KU-501-612

# Nursing the Child with Respiratory Problems

WITHDRAWN

LOTHIAN COLL. HEALTH STUDIES

9
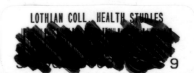

# Nursing the Child with Respiratory Problems

*Joan Ramsay* RGN, DipN(London), Cert Ed, RNT

Senior Tutor
Charles West School of Nursing
Great Ormond Street

LIBRARY
NORTH LOTHIAN COLLEGE
OF NURSING & MIDWIFERY
13 CREWE ROAD SOUTH
EDINBURGH EH4 2LD

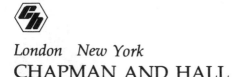

*London   New York*
CHAPMAN AND HALL

618. 922 004 231 RAM

First published in 1989 by
Chapman and Hall Ltd
11 New Fetter Lane, London EC4P 4EE

© 1989 Joan Ramsay

Typeset in 10/12 Palacio by
Mayhew Typesetting, Bristol
Printed in Great Britain by
St. Edmundsbury Press Ltd
Bury St. Edmunds, Suffolk

ISBN  0 412 32410 5

This paperback edition is sold subject to the
condition that it shall not, by way of trade or
otherwise, be lent, resold, hired out, or
otherwise circulated without the publisher's
prior consent in any form of binding or cover
other than that in which it is published and
without a similar condition including this
condition being imposed on the subsequent
purchaser.

All rights reserved. No part of this book may
be reprinted or reproduced, or utilized in any
form or by any electronic, mechanical or other
means, now known or hereafter invented,
including photocopying and recording, or in
any information storage and retrieval system,
without permission in writing from the
publisher.

**British Library Cataloguing in Publication Data**

Ramsay, Joan
  Nursing the child with respiratory problems
  1. Respiratory patients. Children. Nursing
  I. Title
  610.73'62
  ISBN 0–412–32410–5

# Contents

# Preface

This book is primarily intended for RSCN students to use as an introduction or a consolidation to the care of children with respiratory problems. It may also be of value to other nurses and professional staff who are involved in the care of these children.

Respiratory disorders are more common and have potentially more serious consequences in children than in adults. This may be due to congenital malformations or caused by the immature structure and function of the respiratory tract during childhood. To illustrate these points the first two chapters are devoted to the embryology, anatomy and physiology of the respiratory system of the child.

The management of children with respiratory disorders also differs markedly from that of adults. One major difference lies in the observation of the sick child, especially in the young infant who cannot explain how he feels. To help the nurse to appreciate the importance of observing the child with a respiratory illness Chapter 3 explores this aspect. Another variation is found in the treatment given to children with a respiratory problem. Adaptions to the treatment given to adults with respiratory problems must be made because of the child's small size and immaturity. Chapter 4 discusses some of the main differences in respiratory therapy.

The remaining chapters are concerned with the common childhood respiratory disorders. The nursing care is set out using the components of the nursing process – assessment, planning, implementation and evaluation, and is based on Nancy Roper's model of nursing. Each chapter includes a problem-solving care plan for an individual child, of the age most usually affected by each particular disorder. This is intended to illustrate not only the specific care required for that disorder, but also the specific problems encountered when nursing children of different ages. It is important to recognize that the care is related only to the respiratory disorder and does not, for example, include a complete assessment of the child on admission. For convenience, the nurse is referred to as 'she' and the child as 'he' throughout the text.

## ACKNOWLEDGEMENTS

I would like to thank all the staff on Ward 5B, The Hospital for Sick Children, Great Ormond Street, especially Su Madge and Amani Prasad for their advice and support. I am also indebted to my mother who typed the manuscript so efficiently and accurately in spite of her lack of experience with medical terminology.

Joan Ramsay, 1988

# 1 The development of the respiratory system

Some of the disorders of respiration which occur during childhood are due to malformation or abnormalities which occur during fetal development.

The Chinese calculate the age of their children not by the child's date of birth but by the date of conception. Development of the new human being begins from the moment of conception and disorders of the respiratory system can also occur as a result of hereditary or environmental factors.

## 1.1 INHERITANCE

The moment of conception is when the nucleus of the father's sperm fuses with the nucleus of the mother's ovum. The characteristics of the new human being will depend partly on inheritance. Inherited factors are present in minute segments of deoxyribonucleic acid (DNA) called genes. The genes are distributed along microscopic structures known as chromosomes.

Human cells contain 23 pairs of chromosomes. Reproductive cells or gametes are formed by meiotic division during which the 23 pairs of chromosomes are split into two, producing 23 chromatids in each gamete. When the paired chromosomes split they also break and change sections with each other thus altering the genetic information and producing a different effect from before. This change in a gene is known as a mutation. A mutant gene remains unchanged and is transmitted during reproduction. At reproduction fusion of the gametes restores the normal number of 23 pairs of chromosomes. Each pair will consist of one chromatid from the father and one from the mother.

Numerous genetic defects which influence development are

being discovered. The development of the respiratory tract is affected by cystic fibrosis, an inherited disorder caused by the mutation of a gene. There is a familial tendency in asthma that may also be due to genetic factors.

## 1.2 EMBRYONIC DEVELOPMENT

### The first week

Fertilization usually occurs in the uterine tube. Within hours, mitosis of the combined nuclei begins and forms two blastomeres. On the second day following fertilization further division gives rise to the four blastomere stage. This cell division continues until a solid ball of approximately 64 cells, called a morula, has been formed (Figure 1.1). At about this stage the cells begin to differentiate and the morula changes into a blastocyst. The blastocyst is a hollow, fluid-containing ball with an inner and outer mass of cells. The outer cell mass or trophoblast will eventually form part of the placenta and the inner cell mass will become the fetus.

Protusions of the trophoblast burrow into the uterine endometrium so that, by the end of the first week after fertilization, the blastocyst is implanted in the uterine wall.

### The second week

During the second week after fertilization the cells of the inner cell mass differentiate. An embryonic disc forms consisting of two distinct layers: endoderm which produces the yolk sac, and ectoderm which produces the amniotic sac. A fluid-filled split appears between the ectoderm and the inner surface of the trophoblast to form the amniotic cavity.

Cells migrate from the trophoblast to give rise to a third distinct layer of tissue, the primitive mesoderm. Embedded in this layer of mesoderm are two vesicles. By the end of the second week a thickening occurs in the endodermal vesicle. Anteriorly, this thickening is known as the prochordal plate and is the beginning of the development of the mouth (Figure 1.2).

### The third week

During the third week there is a period of rapid embryonic

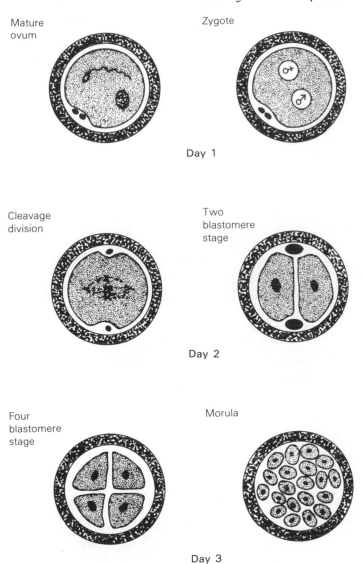

**Figure 1.1** Fertilization and cleavage.

development. This rapid development is made possible by the fact that the embryo can now derive nourishment from and eliminate waste into the maternal circulation.

A thickening of the ectoderm layer forms the primitive streak.

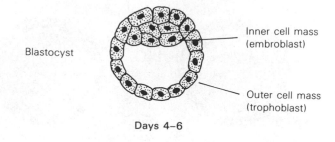

Blastocyst

Inner cell mass (embroblast)

Outer cell mass (trophoblast)

**Days 4–6**

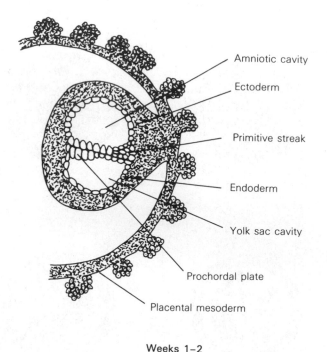

Amniotic cavity

Ectoderm

Primitive streak

Endoderm

Yolk sac cavity

Prochordal plate

Placental mesoderm

**Weeks 1–2**

**Figure 1.2**  Formation of germ layers.

The rounded end of the streak marks the cranial end. At this head end it fuses with the underlying endoderm to form the oropharyngeal membrane. At the caudal end the fusion of ectoderm and endoderm forms the cloacal membrance.

Along the primitive streak secondary mesoderm is formed. At the cranial end of the streak this mesoderm produces the notochordal process which eventually hollows to form a tubular structure, the notochordal canal.

The three layers of ectoderm, mesoderm and endoderm that are now present will form the basis of all the tissues and organs of the developing baby. The ectoderm forms the surface of the body (skin, hair and nails), the epithelial lining of organs (nose, mouth and anus) and the nervous system. The mesoderm layer develops into muscle, bone, connective tissue, blood vessels and cells and the urogenital system. The endoderm forms most of the inner organs; the gastrointestinal organs and the organs of the respiratory system.

## The fourth week

By the end of the third week the notochord develops from the notochordal canal. The notochord is the beginning of the development of the nervous system and is the basis for the formation of the vertebral canal (Figure 1.3).

Also at this stage the mesoderm splits into segments (somites). The somites eventually form the axial skeleton. At the beginning of the fourth week the embryo is almost straight

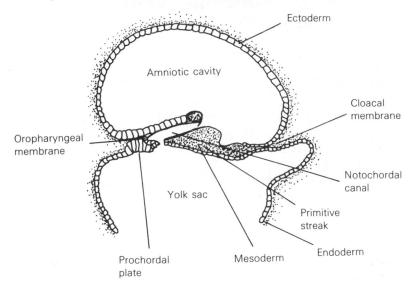

Weeks 3–4

**Figure 1.3** Early embryonic development.

with somites producing bulges along its sides. It grows more rapidly in length than in width and as a result it folds to become a cylindrical curved embryo. As the embryo continues to curve the prochordal plate becomes the cranial end of the foregut. The ectoderm joins it to form the stomodeum or primitive oral cavity. The larger cranial end of the foregut becomes the pharynx.

Spaces in the mesoderm either side of the somites fuse to form the intraembryonic coelom – a horseshoe-shaped cavity. This is the beginning of the development of the peritardium, pleura and peritoneum.

From this stage to the eighth week following fertilization all the major structures and organs of the body start to develop. It is at this stage that the embryo is most at risk from developmental damage by teratogens.

## 1.3 DEVELOPMENT OF THE UPPER RESPIRATORY TRACT

### The nose and mouth

Development of the face takes place mainly between the fifth and eighth week after fertilization. The mesoderm around the stomodeum (mouth) thickens in five places. One of these areas of hypertrophy, the frontonasal prominence, is the beginning of the development of the nose.

At the beginning of the fifth week the mesoderm on either side of the frontonasal process forms two C-shaped areas, the medial and lateral nasal prominences (Figure 1.4). In the centre of each prominence are two nasal pits. As both nasal prominences develop the nasal pits deepen to form nasal sacs or cavities. The inferior turbinate bones develop from the lateral wall of these cavities. At this time the nasal cavities are separated from the stomodeum by the baccalnasal membrane. This membrane disappears during the seventh week to allow communication between the nose and mouth. The mesoderm lining the roof of the nasal cavities develops into olfactory epithelium and becomes sensitive to smell. Nerve fibres from this specialized epithelium extend to the cerebrum to transmit smell.

Occasionally there may be a congenital absence of the nose, with or without an aperture. Acquired deformities, such as the imperfect development of the nasal bones, once a common result

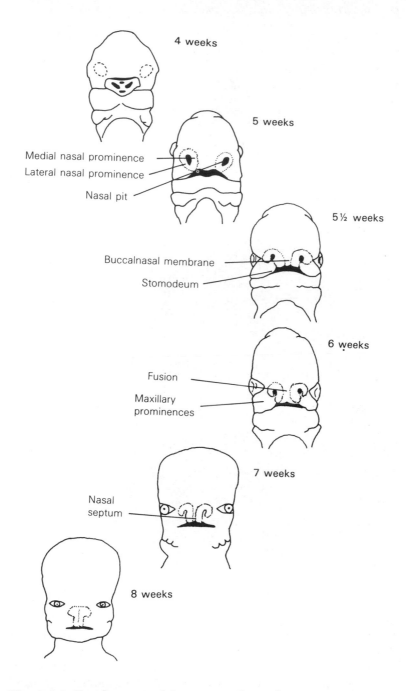

**Figure 1.4** Development of the nose and mouth.

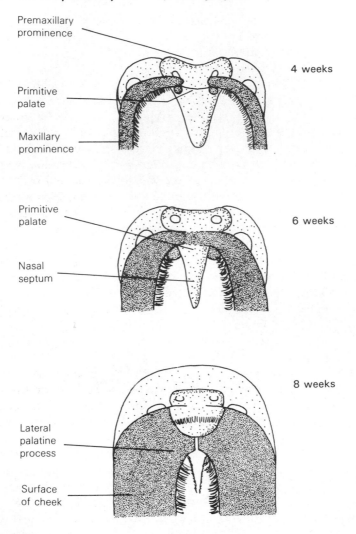

Premaxillary prominence

Primitive palate

Maxillary prominence

4 weeks

Primitive palate

Nasal septum

6 weeks

8 weeks

Lateral palatine process

Surface of cheek

**Figure 1.5** Development of the palate.

of congenital syphilis, are more often seen. Probably the most important congenital defect involving the nose is choanal atresia. Undiagnosed choanal atresia can lead to neonatal anoxia and death. This defect, often associated with a wide variety of anomalies, is caused by the buccalnasal membrane remaining in place. At birth babies instinctively breathe through the nose and have to learn to mouth breathe. Neonates with nasal obstruction such as choanal atresia are therefore cyanosed and dyspnoeic. This condition is made worse by an activity which includes the oropharynx, for example, sucking and feeding. Prompt diagnosis and the establishment of an airway is essential.

During the sixth and seventh week the medial nasal prominences fuse with the mesoderm between the maxillae to form the nasal septum and the middle of the upper lip. This intermaxillary part also forms the primitive palate (Figure 1.5). During the ninth week the primitive palate joins with the nasal septum and the lateral palatine processes which develop from the two maxillary prominences around the stomadeum.

The primitive palate ossifies and bone also develops at the front of the lateral palatine processes to form the hard palate. The remaining area posteriorly is the soft palate and uvula.

In about one in 2500 births the palatine processes fail to join with the primitive palate and the nasal septum. A cleft palate results. This failure of development is often due to maternal drugs, such as steroids. These babies are at risk from respiratory infection as feeds can be regurgitated through the nose.

### The throat

During the fourth week after fertilization three pairs of branchial arches develop beside the pharynx. The first of these arches will eventually form the head and neck. Each branchial arch consists of cartilage, muscle, a nerve and an artery. The first arch ossifies to form the mandible and the cartilage of the second and third arches develop into the hyoid bone.

Four pairs of pharyngeal pouches are formed from the endoderm lining the pharynx as the branchial arches develop. The palatine tonsil develops from the second pouch (Figure 1.6).

Congenital abnormalities caused by maldevelopment of the branchial arches are comparatively rare. The most common is Pierre Robin syndrome (micrognathia) where, among other abnormalities of the face, the mandible is so small and the tongue relatively large, that feeding is difficult and sometimes respiration is impaired.

### The larynx and trachea

At the beginning of the fifth week following fertilization a cleft or respiratory diverticulum develops at the base of the posterior

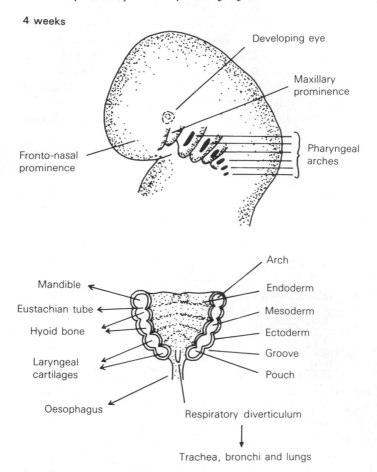

4 weeks

Developing eye

Maxillary
prominence

Pharyngeal
arches

Fronto-nasal
prominence

Arch

Mandible

Endoderm

Eustachian tube

Mesoderm

Hyoid bone

Ectoderm

Groove

Laryngeal
cartilages

Pouch

Oesophagus

Respiratory diverticulum

Trachea, bronchi and lungs

**Figure 1.6**  Development of the throat.

end of the pharynx. Tracheo-oesophageal folds grow inwards
along the edges of the cleft to split that part of the foregut. The
two parts thus formed are the oesophagus and the laryngotracheal tube. The lining of these structures is composed of endoderm which develops into the epithelial lining and glands of the
lower respiratory tract. Also at this time three swellings develop
which grow into the respiratory diverticulum. As a result the
orifice becomes Y-shaped. The anterior swelling develops into
the epiglottis and the lateral swellings form the laryngeal
cartilages (Figure 1.7). The epithelial tissue is, at this stage, grow-
ing so rapidly that it actually occludes the developing larynx. The

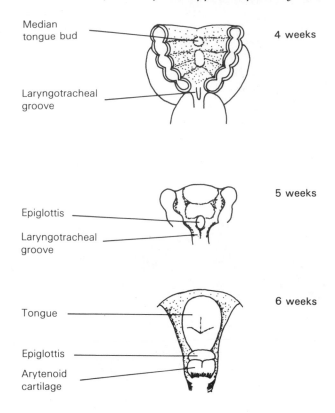

Median tongue bud

Laryngotracheal groove

4 weeks

Epiglottis

Laryngotracheal groove

5 weeks

Tongue

Epiglottis

Arytenoid cartilage

6 weeks

**Figure 1.7**   Development of the larynx.

largynx reopens during the tenth week and is strengthened by rings of cartilage which have developed from the fourth and sixth branchial arches.

The laryngotracheal tube elongates as the embryo grows to form the larynx and trachea. The cranial part of the respiratory diverticulum becomes the larynx and opens into the laryngo-pharynx. The caudal end of the diverticulum forms the buds of the developing lungs.

A rare congenital defect is a laryngeal web. This occurs when a fold of epithelium remains across the larynx after the tenth week. Diagnosis is usually made during the first year of life due to a stridor. If the abnormality is not recognized at this early stage, the child usually presents with a difficulty in speech.

In about one in every 2500 births the tracheo–oesophageal folds do not unite to form a septum between the oesophagus

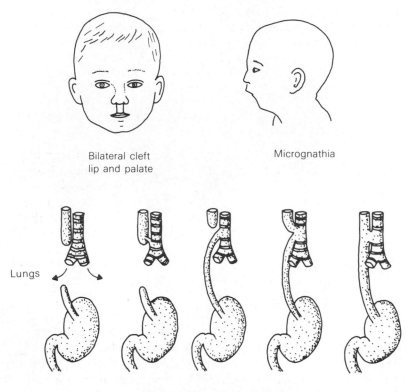

Bilateral cleft
lip and palate

Micrognathia

Lungs

Types of oesophageal atresia
and tracheo-oesophageal fistula

**Figure 1.8** Malformations of the palate and trachea.

and laryngotracheal tube. A trachea–oesophageal fistula
results. Sometimes stenosis of the trachea or oesophageal
atresia are associated malformations (Figure 1.8). When the
baby is fed, milk either flows directly into the trachea or spills
over into it. Gastric contents in the lung can cause pneomonitis
and air entering the abdominal cavity causes distension.

Congenital tracheal stenosis can occur. The degree of stenosis
is variable and is caused by abnormally numerous and complete
rings of cartilage either affecting a short segment or the
complete length of the trachea. If the degree of stenosis is
severe the neonate will have a harsh stridor and dyspnoea.
Stridor may also be a feature of tracheomalacia. This rare
congenital problem is due to abnormal flaccidity of the trachea

of unknown cause. The flaccidity allows the superstructure of the trachea to be driven in by the incoming air, giving a very small entry into the bronchi. It is very rarely associated with absence of the cartilaginous rings.

## 1.4 DEVELOPMENT OF THE LOWER RESPIRATORY TRACT

### The bronchi and lungs

During the fifth week of embryonic development the lung buds which have formed at the caudal end of the respiratory diverticulum begin to divide. Up until the sixteenth week they subdivide repeatedly to form the bronchial tree. As the lung buds develop and grow into the primitive pleural cavity, the surrounding mesoderm forms the visceral pleura. At this stage the ultimate branches end blindly and the lungs have a glandular appearance (Figure 1.9). Although the branches are lined by cuboidal epithelium and are surrounded by capillaries, there is not yet any means for gaseous exchange.

After the sixteenth week further subdivisions take place to form the terminal bronchioles and the alveolar ducts. Some primitive alveoli also appear and the area becomes more vascular. By about 20 weeks these changes allow for some respiratory movement to occur and an exchange of alveoli fluid takes place in the alveoli.

From about 24 weeks up until term the lungs of the fetus develop further. The number of alveoli increases rapidly and the epithelium flattens to become squamous. Capillaries make up most of the lung surface. By the time the fetus is 24–28 weeks old the lungs have matured sufficiently to allow independent respiration if born prematurely. At about 24–28 weeks the alveolar walls secrete a detergent called surfactant. Surfactants are lipids which reduce the surface tension of fluid covering the surfaces of the alveoli. This reduction of tension counteracts the elastic resistance of the lungs to expansion and allows the alveoli to distend with the baby's first breath at birth. Surfactants also help to keep the alveoli distended between breaths.

Babies who are born prematurely and have immature lungs with a lack of surfactant often cannot initiate or continue respiration. This is known as respiratory distress syndrome (RDS). Such babies need continuous positive airway pressure to prevent alveolar collapse.

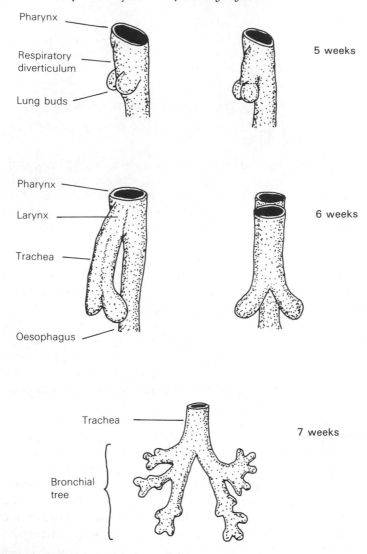

**Figure 1.9** Development of the bronchi and lungs.

Abnormalities in the development of the lungs can occur.
Bilateral and unilateral agenesis of the lungs can occur.
Unilateral agenesis of the lung is usually incompatible with a
normal life expectancy partly due to associated malformations
and partly due to pulmonary infection. Occasionally the lung
buds subdivide haphazardly to produce an accessory lung or

lobe. These accessory structures do not usually communicate with the vascular system or the bronchi and therefore are symptomless. Pulmonary sequestrations (masses of pulmonary tissue which do not connect with the tracheobronchial tree and receive blood from systemic arteries) can occur within or separate from the lung but are usually also asymptomatic.

If space in part of the thorax is restricted, for instance, when abdominal organs have herniated into the thorax from a defect in the diaphragm, hypoplasia of the associated lung will occur. When this happens the other lung often hypertrophies to compensate causing a mediastinal shift. Bilateral lung hypoplasia can occur but is usually associated with hypoplasia of other organs.

Some types of lung cysts are congenital. Anomalous lung buds in the laryngotracheal tube develop into bronchogenic cysts and cause narrowing and obstruction of the oesophagus or one of the major bronchi. Peripheral cysts of the bronchi can form at a later stage of fetal development. These cysts trap inspired air as soon as independent respiration commences after birth. As a result they either expand rapidly and cause displacement of other thoracic organs or they rupture into the pleural cavity to cause a tension pneumothorax.

The development of the lungs continues after birth until about eight years of age. For the first three years of life primitive alveoli and bronchioles continue to develop until they have increased their number sevenfold. From three to eight years maturation of these primitive structures occurs. Once maturation has occurred no further alveoli can develop.

## The diaphragm

At the end of the third week the embryonic heart occupies the whole width of the body. It is separated from the liver by a thick layer of mesoderm, the septum transversum, which develops to form the central tendon, the diaphragm (Figure 1.10).

During the fifth week the development of the lungs and pleura widens the thorax. At the same time the developing liver widens the abdomen. The body wall between the pleural and peritoneal cavities is drawn inwards to form the domes of the diaphragm. The mesentery around the dorsal part of the oesophagus forms the central part of the diaphragm. The

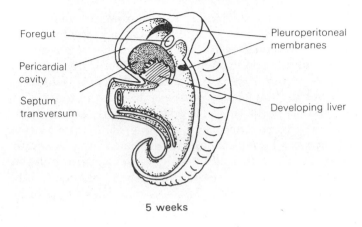

Foregut

Pleuroperitoneal membranes

Pericardial cavity

Septum transversum

Developing liver

5 weeks

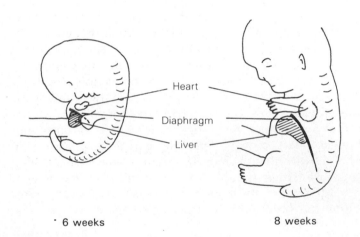

Heart

Diaphragm

Liver

6 weeks

8 weeks

**Figure 1.10**  Development of the diaphragm.

diaphragm is completed at the end of the fifth week by the pleuroperitoneal membranes. These membranes develop from the body wall and fuse with the oesophageal mesentery and the septum transversum.

In about 1 in every 2000 births this fusion is incomplete resulting in a congenital diaphragmatic hernia. Abdominal organs herniate into the thorax displacing the heart and mediastinum. The lungs become compressed and their growth is retarded causing respiratory distress at birth.

# 2 The anatomy and physiology of the respiratory system during childhood

Some of the most common health problems during childhood are related to disturbances of respiratory function. The immature structure of the respiratory tract during childhood often makes the child more susceptible to respiratory disorders and also to react to the disorder more severely than an adult.

At birth the respiratory system is relatively small. Although fetal respiratory movements can be seen at about 20 weeks and exchange of amniotic fluids occurs in the alveoli, the placenta is responsible for gaseous exchange. At birth chemical and thermal stimuli initiate the first breath and the alveoli become responsible for the exchange of oxygen and carbon dioxide. After this first breath the lungs grow rapidly, especially during the first year of life. In spite of this rapid growth during infancy the respiratory system is not completely mature until the age of about eight years.

The respiratory system is composed of all the structures involved in the passage of air from the nose to the alveoli. The upper part of the tract from the nose to the larynx is not involved in gaseous exchange and, for this reason, is often termed the 'dead space'. The lower respiratory tract which is actively involved in the exchange of gases comprises the structures from the trachea to the aveoli (Figure 2.1).

NORTH LOTHIAN COLLEGE OF NURSING LIBRARY

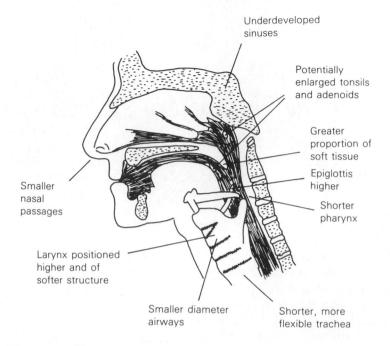

Underdeveloped
sinuses

Potentially
enlarged tonsils
and adenoids

Greater
proportion of
soft tissue

Epiglottis
higher

Shorter
pharynx

Smaller
nasal
passages

Larynx positioned
higher and of
softer structure

Smaller diameter
airways

Shorter, more
flexible trachea

**Figure 2.1**  The respiratory tract of the child.

## 2.1 THE UPPER RESPIRATORY TRACT

### The nose

On inspiration air is first passed into the nose. In the infant the
nasal passages are small as the absence of teeth means that the
jaws are underdeveloped. Consequently, the nose can easily
become blocked by secretions. As infants are unable to use their
mouths for breathing any obstruction of the nose may be
hazardous.

The outer nose is composed of a bony framework surrounding a large irregular cavity. This cavity is divided into two equal
parts by a bony and cartilaginous septum. In children the
septum may be prolonged backwards. Examination of the
vestibule of the nose in a child must therefore consist of
pushing the tip of the nose upwards whilst tilting the child's
head backwards.

In the bones of the face and cranium are air-filled cavities
called sinuses. The sinuses connect with the nasal cavities by

means of small openings. The sinuses add resonance to the voice and lighten the bones of the cranium.

In the child the sinuses are not well developed. Sinus development in the fetus does not begin until the end of pregnancy when diverticula grow out from the lateral walls of the nasal cavities. The maxillary sinuses, which are only a few millimetres across at birth, do not grow to adult size until late adolescence when all the permanent teeth are present. The ethmoidal sinuses, which are also small at birth, develop during the first ten years of life. The frontal and sphenoidal sinuses do not develop at all until the age of two. At about the this time the anterior pair of ethmoid sinuses grow into the frontal bone to form the frontal sinuses, and the posterior pair enter the sphenoid bone to form the sphenoidal sinuses.

The nose is linked with a very vascular ciliated epithelium. Its vascularity warms the air as it passes over the interior nasal surface. This vascularity also means that episodes of epistaxis are common during childhood. Any trauma such as blows to the head, nose picking or foreign bodies inserted into the nose may cause bleeding to occur readily. Bleeding may also be associated with inflammation of the nasal mucosa due to an infection of the upper respiratory tract. Childhood epistaxis usually stops spontaneously and does not require medical intervention.

**The pharynx**

The nose opens into the pharynx via the posterior nares. The pharynx, a muscular tube 12–14 cm long, extends from the base of the skull to the level of the sixth cervical vertebra in adults but is shorter in the child. For the first year of life the infant's pharynx is 8–10 cm long and extends to the level of the fourth cervical vertebra.

The auditory tubes connect the nasal part of the pharynx with the middle ears. In early childhood middle ear infection is commonly a complication of respiratory infections as the causative organism can easily spread via this route.

The pharyngeal tonsils or adenoids, which consist of a mass of lymphoid tissue, lie on the posterior wall of the nasopharynx between the two auditory tubes and opposite the posterior nares. They filter and protect the respiratory and alimentary tracts from pathogenic organisms. They are not present in adulthood as gradual atrophy takes place after the age of seven years. Occasionally the adenoids are grossly swollen, not always due to chronic infection. Enlargement causes partial obstruction of the airways, the infant develops noisy breathing and the older child begins to mouth breathe which predisposes him to further infection, and snores at night. Enlarged adenoids may also block the auditory tubes and drainage from the middle ear is impaired resulting in otitis media.

The palatine tonsils are a pair of tonsils which lie in the oral part of the pharynx. These collections of lymphoid tissue are positioned behind and below the soft palate. Their funcåton, like the pharyngeal tonsils, is protection and they also tend to be larger during childhood when respiratory infection is more likely. When these tonsils enlarge due to infection they can meet in the midline and obstruct the passage of air and food. The treatment of chronic tonsillitis by tonsillectomy is not successful before the age of three years as the lympoid tissue often redevelops.

**The larynx**

The larynx lies in front of the laryngopharynx and extends from the origin of the tongue to the trachea. During childhood it is funnel shaped and is composed of a series of irregular shaped cartilages. The first and most prominent of these is the thyroid cartilage which consists of two flat pieces of cartilage which fuse together anteriorly to form the laryngeal prominence or 'Adam's apple'. In adults the thyroid cartilage is incomplete posteriorly but during infancy the two parts are connected by a narrow intra-thyroid cartilage. Immediately below the thyroid cartilage is the cricoid cartilage and attached to that are the two arytenoid cartilages. These are all composed of hyaline cartilage during childhood and become ossified during early adulthood.

The softer structure of the larynx and its small diameter in early childhood predisposes the infant and young child to serious airway obstruction when any inflammation of the larynx occurs.

The epiglottis, a U-shaped cartilage in children, is attached to the inferior surface of the thyroid cartilage. During swallowing it occludes the laryngopharyngeal opening to prevent food and liquid passing into the trachea. In infancy the tip of the epiglottis is situated just above the thyroid cartilage and lies

level with the area between the odontoid process and the body
of the axis. This relatively high position makes the epiglottis
vulnerable to the spread of infection from the nose and throat.
When it becomes inflammed it can cause laryngeal obstruction
and death. In adults the tip of the epiglottis is level with the
hyoid bone. Between infancy and adulthood the larynx moves
downwards, a distance of two vertebral bodies and two
intervertebral discs, to lie opposite the fourth, fifth and sixth
cervical vertebrae.

In the male the larynx undergoes further change during
puberty. At this time (between ten and 14 years) testosterone,
secreted by the interstitial cells of the testes, causes enlargement of all the cartilages. The thyroid cartilage in particular
becomes more prominent and the length of the glottis is almost
doubled. The enlargement of the arytenoid cartilages affects the
vocal cords which lengthen to produce the male's deep voice.

**The trachea**

The trachea is a continuation of the larynx. It is composed of C-
shaped cartilages which are extremely elastic during childhood.
These incomplete rings of cartilage surround two-thirds of the
trachea. The posterior one-third of the trachea and the areas
between the cartilage rings are made up of involuntary muscle
and connective tissue.

In the adult the trachea is about 10–11 cm long and
terminates at about the level of the fifth thoracic vertebra where
it divides into the right and left bronchi. During childhood the
trachea is smaller, approximately 8–9 cm long, and ends on a
level with the fourth thoracic vertebra. It also lies more deeply
and is more flexible than in the adult.

Introducers are often used to intubate children to overcome
this flexibility of the trachea. Plastic and silastic has become the
preferred material for paediatric tracheostomy tubes as they
conform to the contours of the trachea.

## 2.2 THE LOWER RESPIRATORY TRACT

**The bronchi**

The trachea divides into two main bronchi. The right bronchus
is wider, shorter and more vertical than the left bronchus. As

it lies more directly below the trachea than the left side, inhaled foreign bodies are more likely to fall to the right. The right bronchus also differs from the left at its entry to the lungs. The right bronchus enters the hilum of the right lung at about the level of the fourth thoracic vertebra during childhood. The left bronchus enters the hilum of the left lung at the level of the fifth thoracic vertebra. During childhood the bronchi lengthen and by adulthood they enter the lungs at the level of the fifth and sixth vertebrae respectively.

The relative shortness of the respiratory tract during early childhood means that any infection of the upper respiratory tract easily spreads to all areas.

**The lungs**

On entering the lungs the bronchi subdivide into lobar bronchi and segmental bronchi. At this stage the plates of cartilage which make up this structure disappear and subsequent subdivisions are known as bronchioles. The bronchioles subdivide about ten times eventually leading to the alveoli. Although the bronchial tree is fully developed at birth the number of alveoli continues to increase until about the age of three years. From the age of three they also grow in size as the chest develops and continue to do so until the lungs reach adult proportions. Obviously the development of the lungs is closely related to body size and the shape of the chest as the child grows. As the lungs develop they become more efficient; the expired air contains less oxygen and more carbon dioxide (Table 2.1).

At birth the lungs are pinkish-white but become mottled with grey with age and by adulthood they are a dark grey colour. The initial breath after birth is initiated partly by chemical and partly by thermal stimuli. The chemical stimuli are the low oxygen, high carbon dioxide level and low pH of the blood which triggers the respiratory centre in the medulla. The respiratory centre is also stimulated by sensory impulses in the skin which are excited by the sudden cooling of the baby as he leaves the relatively warm environment of the uterus.

Air entry initially is obstructed by the amniotic fluid in the fetal lungs and alveoli. At birth some of this fluid is removed by the pulmonary capillaries and lymphatics. The rest of the fluid is squeezed out due to the pressure on the baby's thorax

**Table 2.1** A comparison of blood chemistry between the newborn and the adult

| | Arterial blood chemistry | |
| --- | --- | --- |
| | At birth | After birth |
| $pO_2$ | 65–80 mmHg | 85–105 mmHg |
| $pCO_2$ | 27–40 mmHg | 32–45 mmHg |
| pH | 7.3 | 7.4 |

as he passes through the birth canal. Once the chest has been delivered the brisk recoil of the thorax allows air to enter to replace the lost fluid.

The alveoli retain some air even at the end of expiration so each subsequent breath requires less effort. Pneumocytes in the alveolar epithelium secrete a protein surfactant. This fluid prevents the collapsed alveoli from drying out and also stops the fall in pressure which occurs when the lungs expand during inspiration.

Without surfactant, as in premature babies, the alveoli collapse completely between each breath. Each respiration requires the same effort as the initial breath and leads to exhaustion and sometimes respiratory failure.

## 2.3 THE THORACIC CAVITY

The thoracic cavity is made up of 12 thoracic vertebrae, 12 pairs of ribs and the sternum. At birth the thoracic cavity is round due to the horizontal position of the ribs. In the adult the ribs join the thoracic vertebrae and sternum at a downward and lateral angle. During inspiration the intercostal muscles contract lifting the ribs to a horizontal position and increasing the chest cavity.

The chest cavity remains more or less round until the age of three or four years. At this age the chest cavity flattens both anteriorly and posteriorly. Until this flattening occurs respiration is mainly a result of a movement of the muscles of the diaphragm and abdomen as contraction of the intercostal muscles would only raise the ribs further and decrease the chest cavity. Instead, chest expansion during inspiration is achieved by relaxation of the abdominal muscles and contraction of the diaphragmatic muscles. These muscle movements force the diaphragm downwards.

The change in the angle of the articulation of the ribs with the sternum and the thoracic vertebrae is largely due to the gradual ossification of the sternum as the child grows. At birth the posterior part of the sternum is entirely cartilaginous. Ossification of this region occurs during the first three years of life.

In the adult the sternum consists of three parts, the manubrium, gladiolus and ensiform cartilage. The gladiolus consists of five segments which do not fuse until puberty.

# 3 The assessment of the child with a respiratory problem

Nursing children with respiratory problems has the same aims as any type of nursing. Those aims are to help children to reach an optimum level of health, to overcome illness or to adjust and cope with their problems. In order to meet these aims effectively the nurse must be able to make an accurate assessment of each child. This assessment involves the collection of information using interview techniques, observation and physical examination. Assessment is usually performed when the nurse first meets the child but should be continuous so that the nurse is aware of any changes that may occur. The information collected may help to confirm a diagnosis when this has not yet been positively made. Laboratory investigations are also part of assessment as they aid in the confirmation of a diagnosis. The nurse is involved in caring for children before, during and after these investigations to ensure that the results are accurate and that the child comes to no harm.

Thus, the four components of assessment are:

- history taking from child and parents
- observation of the child
- physical examination
- laboratory investigation

To collect the necessary information during the assessment of a child with a respiratory problem the nurse firstly needs to have an understanding of the normal respiratory system, respiration and the factors which influence breathing in health.

## 3.1 FACTORS AFFECTING BREATHING IN HEALTH

Many factors may affect breathing even in the healthy child. The age of the child and the stage of development will affect his respiration. Physical, psychological, social and environmental factors also alter breathing in various ways (Table 3.1).

**Table 3.1** Factors that affect respiration

Overcrowding
Emotion
Smoking
Climate
Activity
Person's size
Pollution

### The age and development of the child

The rate of respiration varies with the age of the child. The need for oxygen diminishes as metabolic rate and growth decrease with age. Consequently the infant and young child have comparatively high respiratory rates but by the age of about eight years the rate is similar to that of an adult (Table 3.2).

**Table 3.2** Average respiratory rates of children at rest

| Age | Respiratory rate/min |
|---|---|
| Newborn | 50 |
| 3 months | 40 |
| 6 months | 35 |
| 1 year | 30 |
| 2 years | 25 |
| 4 years | 23 |
| 6 years | 21 |
| 8 years | 20 |
| 10–12 years | 18 |
| 13–16 years | 16 |

Up to the age of six months the infant has not developed the ability to cough so this will not be a feature of any respiratory illness at this age. In older children, particularly those between one and two years who delight in mimicking, coughing may merely be a means of attracting attention rather than an indication of illness.

## Physical factors

At birth the neonate's respiration is a guide to the adequacy of ventilation. If the infant has no difficulty in adjusting to extrauterine life his breathing will be regular and between 40 and 60 breaths/min. Six to eight hours after birth the neonate enters a 'period of reactivity'. During this time he is intensely active and the respiratory rate can rise as high as 82 breaths/min. This increase in ventilation aids in the excretion of respiratory mucus. After this active phase the infant settles and respiration decreases.

During play or exercise the respiratory rate increases and, conversely, during rest it decreases. Comparisons of respiratory rate are only completely accurate if the child is at the same level of activity during each recording.

## Psychological factors

The child's emotions affect the respiratory rate. Although a good cry immediately after birth indicates good ventilation, crying increases the respiratory rate and makes accurate measurement impossible.

Suddenly approaching an infant can sometimes startle him and cause an increase in his respiratory rate. This increased respiratory rate caused by stimulation of the sympathetic nervous system can also be due to extreme happiness if the infant or child is playing and gurgling or singing. Children who are anxious may also breathe faster.

A slow respiratory rate is found in infants and young children who are lethargic sometimes due to emotional deprivation. Older children who are sad or depressed will also have a decreased respiratory rate.

**Social factors**

Poor housing conditions may affect the respiratory system. Overcrowded conditions predispose the child to respiratory infections as many more micro-organisms are sprayed into the air during breathing and talking. These organisms also multiply more readily in the warm, moist, stagnant atmosphere created by overcrowding.

Smoking is a cultural practice which has acquired popularity in the UK during the last hundred years. Tobacco smoke is composed of tiny droplets of tar which, when inhaled, penetrate the defences of the lungs. According to the Royal College of Physicians' 1977 report, a non-smoker in the company of smokers may inhale as much smoke as an average smoker inhales from one cigarette. There is some evidence that children whose parents are smokers have a higher incidence of bronchiolitis and pneumonia. Harlop and Davies (1974) found that babies whose mothers smoked were at greater risk of admission to hospital for the treatment of bronchitis or pneumonia. Colley *et al.* (1973) demonstrated that school-age children of smokers were at greater risk of respiratory tract infection.

**Environmental factors**

*Climate*

Children under the age of five have an immature hypothalamus and have difficulty maintaining body temperature. In extremes of environmental temperature they are liable to heat exhaustion or hypothermia. Rising temperatures cause an increase in metabolic rate and thus respiratory rate. Eventually heat exhaustion and respiratory distress will occur. Loss of body heat causes a fall in metabolic rate and respirations.

*Pollution*

Children living in cities are exposed to atmospheric pollution from smoke. Inhalation of smoke, which results from combustion of materials in heating systems, industrial processes and road vehicles, irritates the mucous membrane linings of the respiratory tract. In a damp climate, condensation and smoke produce fog which exacerbates the problem. Prolonged irritation of respiratory tissues predisposes the affected child to respiratory tract infections.

An increased incidence of respiratory tract infections may also be caused by pollution in the home. Inadequate ventilation with increased temperature and humidity predisposes to an increase in the number of microorganisms in the air. Inhalation of gases from faulty heating appliances can cause depression of respirations.

## 3.2 HISTORY TAKING

A nursing history of a child with a respiratory disorder is primarily concerned with the collection of information which will enable the nurse to appreciate the child's usual behaviour and activities in relation to breathing and to identify any particular problems which need nursing intervention. The first activity of life is breathing. It is a vital activity as it provides oxygen for all the cells of the body. Consequently, all other activities of living are dependent on the ability to breathe, and any disorder of breathing may cause an impairment of other body functions. Nancy Roper's 'Model of Nursing' which incorporates 12 activities of daily living is, therefore, the model to use for this part of the child's assessment (Table 3.3). The aim of history taking, using this model, is to discover:

- usual routines
- what the child can and cannot do for himself
- problems and coping mechanisms
- potential problems

**Table 3.3** Activities of daily living from a model for nursing (Roper, 1976)

| | |
|---|---|
| Maintaining a safe environment | Controlling body temperature |
| Communicating | Mobilizing |
| Breathing | Working and playing |
| Eating and drinking | Expressing sexuality |
| Eliminating | Sleeping |
| Personal cleansing and dressing | Dying |

## Maintaining a safe environment

The most important information will relate to the child's ability to maintain his own airway. To ascertain if the child is infectious and to maintain the safety of others in the ward, it is also important to eliminate the possibility of an infectious illness. Useful questions may be:

- Can the child breathe without artificial support?
- Does he have periods of apnoea or cyanosis? When do these episodes occur?
- Has the child been in contact with any respiratory infection?

Knowledge of the child's home environment may help the nurse to discover if there are any predisposing factors.

## Communicating

Shortness of breath can affect the ability to talk. It may require the nurse to phrase her questions so that the child can answer with the minimum of effort. If possible the nurse needs to explore the child's understanding of his problem. The parents' understanding is also useful; it may reveal feelings of guilt, for example if the illness is inherited or an infection.

- Does the breathing problem hamper the child's communication?
- Hoes does the child and his parents feel about the illness?
- What do the child and his parents understand about the illness?

## Breathing

The nurse should endeavour to find out as much as possible about the actual respiratory disorder and its characteristics.

- Does the child have a problem with breathing? What exactly is the problem?
- What makes breathing easier or more difficult?
- What does the child's normal breathing sound like?
- What is the child's usual colour?
- Does the child have a cough? Is the cough dry or does the child cough up secretions? What makes the cough worse or better?

- What do the secretions look like?
- Is there any pain associated with breathing or coughing? How is this eased?

## Maintaining body temperature

Any respiratory tract infection usually causes a pyrexia which may occur at a particular time of the day. Infants are prone to febrile convulsions if their temperature rises above 39°C. So it is important to discover if this is a problem.

- Does the child appear feverish at any time of day?

## Eating and drinking

Breathlessness always interferes with normal eating and drinking as the mouth is often used as an alternative means of breathing. Infants cannot suck when they are breathless. The presence of copious sputum affects taste and often causes anorexia.

- Does the breathing problem cause an alteration in eating and drinking? In what way?

## Mobilizing

Any dyspnoea will affect the child's usual mobility. In order to plan care and assess the degree of breathlessness, the nurse should discover exactly what exertion makes the child short of breath.

- Is the child's normal level of mobility affected by his respiratory problem? In what way?

## Working and playing

Altered mobility may also affect the child's ability to play. He may now be happier just resting or playing a quiet game. Missing school due to illness may be a concern especially if the child is approaching important examinations. The child's illness may have forced the parents to take time off work. This loss of earnings may add to their concerns.

- Has the child's usual play routine been affected by his illness? How has it altered?

- How has the illness affected the child's schooling?
- Have the parents had to take time off work due to the child's illness? Is this a problem?

## Resting and sleeping

Dyspnoea may make it difficult for the child to rest or sleep unless in an upright position. If the child is struggling to breathe, his consequent exhaustion may cause him to sleep more. Coughing may disturb the rest and sleep of the child and his parents. Parents who are tired may be less able to cope with an ill child.

- Does the child's respiratory problem interfere with his own or his parents' usual pattern of rest and sleep? How?

## Dying

Dyspnoea is always frightening to both the sufferer and the onlookers. Because of this the older child and his parents may have fears that the illness is fatal. The child may have a problem that is known to cause death. The nurse needs a good rapport with the child and his parents to discover if they are worried about death. Talking about their understanding of the illness may help to reveal this.

- Does the child or his parents have any particular fears?

## 3.3 OBSERVATION

Observation of the child's breathing and related problems should occur initially to assess the child's condition and thereafter to evaluate response to treatment. The rate, rhythm, depth and character of respirations must be observed as well as the characteristics of any pain, cough or sputum.

Respirations should be observed before disturbing the child. Infants may cry when handled making accurate recordings impossible; older children who are aware of being watched may immediately change their breathing patterns. A knowledge of the changes which occur in disorders of the respiratory system aids in the interpretation of the observations (Table 3.4).

**Table 3.4** Interpretation of observations of respiration and related problems

| Observation | Abnormality | Possible significance | Rationale |
|---|---|---|---|
| Respiratory rate | Bradypnoea | Cerebral tumour, oversedation or opiate poisoning | Depression of the respiratory centre in the medulla |
| | Tachypnoea | Meningitis, pneumonia, pleurisy | Infection increases the metabolic rate |
| | | Shock, heart failure, anaemia, alkalosis, salicylate poisoning | Lack of circulating oxygen due to defect in circulatory system |
| | Apnoea | Asphyxia (short periods can be normal in neonates) | Obstruction of respiratory tract |
| Depth of respirations | Hyperpnoea | Metabolic acidosis | Excess carbon dioxide |
| | Shallow breathing | Alkalosis, broken ribs, pleurisy | To avoid pain |
| Respiratory rhythm | Periodic (Cheyne-Stokes) breathing | Raised intracranial pressure, terminal illness | Decline in respirations causes build-up of carbon dioxide which briefly restimulates breathing |
| | Slowed expiration | Asthma, emphysema | Obstruction of airflow |
| Breathing sounds | Stridor | Inhalation of a foreign body, inflammation of larynx and trachea | Obstruction of the larynx causing prolonged inspiration |
| | Wheeze | Asthma | Airflow obstruction |
| | Stertorous breathing (snoring) | Cerebral injury | Depression of the respiratory centre |
| | 'Rattling' respiration | Infection of respiratory tract, pulmonary oedema | Presence of excess mucus and fluid |

**Table 3.4** contd

| Observation | Abnormality | Possible significance | Rationale |
|---|---|---|---|
| Colour | Cyanosis with dyspnoea | Disease of chest wall, fibrosis of lungs, severe pneumonia | Damaged chest wall or lung tissue impairs chest movement and oxygen intake |
| | Cyanosis without dyspnoea | Drug overdose, right to left vascular shunt | Depression of respiratory centre, mix of oxygenated and deoxygenated blood |
| Chest movements | Use of abdominal muscles in child over 7 years | Inflammation within chest e.g. pleurisy | Respiration is mostly abdominal in young children. In older children due to pain on using chest muscles |
| | Use of costal muscles in child under 7 years | Acute abdomen, e.g. peritonitis | Respirations mainly costal over 7 years. In younger children due to pain on using abdominal muscles |
| | Use of accessory muscles | Air hunger and ensuing respiratory failure | Severe difficulty in air intake using normal muscles of respiration |
| | Suprasternal Subcostal Intracostal } retractions | Air hunger and ensuring respiratory failure | Retraction of chest wall during inspiration with the severe effort |
| Cough | Dry, unproductive | Anxiety. Early stages of infection of respiratory tract | Irritation of respiratory tract |
| | Productive | Infection or inflammation of respiratory tract, cystic fibrosis, pulmonary oedema | To expectorate excess secretions |

| | | | |
|---|---|---|---|
| Sputum | Mucopurulent | Infection of the respiratory tract or chronic nasal infections | Excess mucus and pus from inflammed linings of respiratory tracts |
| | Frothy | Pulmonary oedema | Fluid in the lungs |
| | Tenacious | Asthma, cystic fibrosis | Swelling of mucosal lining of bronchi or inherited exocrine disorder produces excessive thick secretions |
| | Bloodstained | Blood from epistaxia, swallowed blood | Blood has trickled into respiratory tract |
| | | Haemotysis due to TB, cystic fibrosis | Disease process erodes pulmonary vessels |
| | | 'Rusty' due to pneumonia | |
| | Purulent | Infective lung condition – bronchiectasis, lung abcess | Expectoration of pus from inflammed lungs |
| Other factors | Restlessness, apprehension and nasal flaring | On inspiration – tumour or foreign body in trachea or main bronchus<br>On expiration – asthma, bronchitis or emphysema | Air hunger due to obstruction of upper and lower respiratory tract |

## 3.4 PHYSICAL EXAMINATION

On admission other factors may reveal information about the child's respiratory function. The shape of the chest is often deformed by chronic respiratory disorders. In infancy the chest normally tends to be barrel shaped, but in later childhood this

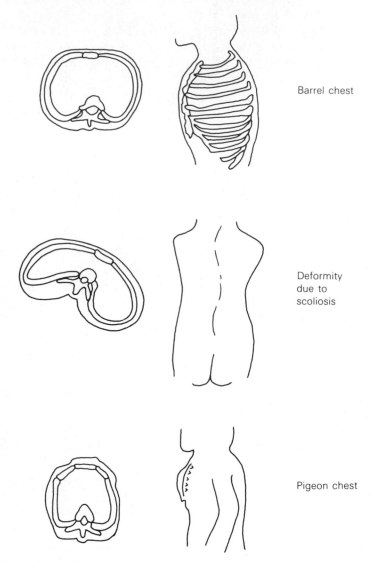

Barrel chest

Deformity
due to
scoliosis

Pigeon chest

**Figure 3.1**  Types of chest deformity.

shape is usually due to long-standing hyperinflation of the lungs due to such chronic problems as asthma, cystic fibrosis or pulmonary emphysema. Chronic chest conditions such as these impair the efficient bellows action of the lungs and because the anatomy of the lungs is distorted, deformity of the thoracic cage occurs. This, in turn, leads to deformities of the spine such as kyphosis and scoliosis.

Pigeon chest, in which the sternum protrudes from the chest wall and there is a series of depressions along the costal-chondral margin ('the ricketty rosary'), is one of the features of rickets (Figure 3.1).

Clubbing of the fingers is a feature of chronic lack of oxygen which can result from respiratory, cardiac or neurological disorders.

When a child with an upper respiratory tract condition is first admitted to hospital, the upper respiratory tract and the ears should be examined. Infection of the lower respiratory system may be due to, or caused by, an upper respiratory infection. The proximity of the middle ear and the throat means that infection is easily transmitted from one structure to the other. Redness of the external ear and swelling of the postauricular and cervical lymph glands indicates an aural infection. The child may show his discomfort by holding or pulling his ears.

Small children dislike keeping their mouth open for examination of the throat so this part of the examination should be kept to last. Using a tongue depresser to view the throat, the tonsils and posterior oropharynx should be clearly visible and, if free of infection, should appear bright pink, smooth, glistening and moist.

## 3.5 INVESTIGATIONS

Although most of the laboratory investigations performed on the respiratory system are carried out by laboratory staff, the nurse has an important role in ensuring that the child remains safe and comfortable throughout any investigative procedure (Table 3.5). The nurse should be able to explain to the child and his parents the purpose of each investigation and what each test involves. These explanations should be in terms that the child and the parents can appreciate. Wherever possible the parents should be able to stay with their child during the test if they wish to do so. The nurse should also remain to show

**Table 3.5** Common respiratory investigations and nursing implications

| Investigation | Definitions and purpose | Nurse's role | | |
|---|---|---|---|---|
| | | Before | During | After |
| Chest X-ray | Films of chest to show deformities | Explain to child and parents | Position child so anterior, posterior and lateral views can be taken. Ensure self or parents have lead apron protection if holding small child | – |
| Lung scan | Inhalation or intravenous injection of radioactive substance to evaluate ventilation or perfusion. Scintillation counters locate and record the density and location of radioactivity | Explain to child and parents | Stay with child | Reassure parents that radioactive substances are quickly eliminated |

## Lung function tests

| | | | | |
|---|---|---|---|---|
| Spirometry | Shows the volumes of air shifted by the lungs | Explain to child and parents | Help laboratory staff to explain breathing pattern necessary | – |
| Vitalography | Measures the forced vital capacity (amount of air that can be forced out following a deep inspiration) | | Ensure child has mouth firmly sealed around mouthpiece | – |
| Peak flow | Shows the fastest air speed achieved during short sharp expiration (peak expiratory flow rate) | Record best of three attempts before drug medication | Ensure child has mouth firmly sealed around mouthpiece | Record best of three attempts following medication |
| Blood gas analysis | Measures oxygen and carbon dioxide content of arterial blood by estimating the pressure exerted by these gases as a part of the total pressure exerted by all blood gases | Explain to child and parents | Expose brachial artery | Maintain pressure on site until bleeding ceases |
| | | | Hold child still | Apply decorative adhesive plaster for older children |

**Table 3.5** contd

| Investigation | Definitions and purpose | Nurse's role | | |
|---|---|---|---|---|
| | | Before | During | After |
| Sputum analysis | To identify specific bacteria or malignant cells, and to find the sensitivity of specific bacteria to antibiotics | Explain to older children the need for material coughed up | Use suction and a sputum trap for babies and younger children | Ensure specimen not kept too long in warm environment of ward |
| Throat and nasal swabs | To identify specific bacteria of malignant cells and to find the sensitivity of specific bacteria to antibiotics | Explain to child and parents | Tip child's head back and take swabs of nasopharynx and oropharynx | Ensure specimen not kept too long in warm environment of ward |
| Cilia function test | Identifies presence of cilia in upper respiratory tract membranes by passage of nasal tube. Biopsy taken by aspirating tube | Explain to child and parents | Stay with child and reassure | – |

| | | | | |
|---|---|---|---|---|
| Sweat test | Diagnoses cystic fibrosis by estimating the amount of sodium and chloride in the sweat. A small electrical current passes pilocarpine into a small area of skin to stimulate local sweat glands | Explain to child and parents<br><br>Expose the thigh for babies and small children, the forearm for older children | After the current has been applied, filter paper, polythene and warm clothing are applied to the area to enhance sweating. These are removed after 20–30 mins | – |
| Bronchoscopy and laryngoscopy | An examination, under general anaesthetic, of the bronchi and larynx by a flexible fibreoptic instrument passed into the mouth | Explain to child and parents<br><br>Starve child for 4–6 h prior to investigation<br><br>Give premedication 1–2 h before theare | – | Observe child for bronchospasm and/or hypoxia<br><br>Ensure child is able to swallow properly before offering food or drink |
| Chest aspiration | Insertion of large-bore needle into pleural space to withdraw fluid and to examine fluid for specific bacteria or malignant cells | Explain to child and parents<br><br>Sedation may be given 1 h before | Sit child upright and support<br><br>Reassure child and parents | Observe for pneumothorax, infection, pulmonary oedema |

them how to hold the child and to reassure them. Following the investigation the nurse should be aware of any potential complications and observe the child for signs of these.

# 4 *Respiratory therapy for children*

Procedures to improve respiratory function are used with increasing frequency to prevent and manage respiratory disorders.

Inhalation therapy includes a variety of therapies which involve the alteration of the composition or volume of inspired air. The inhalation of oxygen increases the oxygen content of inspired air and humidification increases the water vapour content. Drugs can also be added to inspired air and inhaled in the form of airborne particles using an aerosol. Physical therapy involves aiding the normal secretory mechanisms of the lung by using such techniques as deep breathing and coughing exercises, percussion, vibration and postural drainage.

Parents and older children can be taught to perform most of these procedures at home. To practise with confidence, competence and safety they need to be shown not only the techniques involved but also the possible side-effects and any necessary precautions.

## 4.1 OXYGEN THERAPY

Oxygen therapy is employed to relieve hypoxia and to decrease the work of breathing or myocardial activity. There are many different systems for the administration of oxygen to children but the choice of method depends on the concentration of oxygen needed and the child's acceptance of the device. It is important to monitor the concentration of oxygen at least every two hours whichever method is used, as prolonged exposure to oxygen can be damaging to some body tissues. The organs most liable to be damaged are the eyes of premature infants and the lungs of children at any age.

Retrolental fibroplasia is a disease affecting the retina as a result of excessive pressures of oxygen reaching the retinal artery. High oxygen concentrations cause the capillaries in the retina to constrict, and an overgrowth of these developing blood vessels occurs. The hypertrophy of the capillaries causes the retinal veins to multiply and dilate. Retinal oedema, haemorrhaging and detachment results destroying the function of the eye.

Bronchopulmonary dysplasia is a pathological process which occurs in the lungs of babies with respiratory distress syndrome due to high concentrations of oxygen. Excessive oxygen damages the epithelial linings of the bronchioles and causes thickening and fibrosis of the walls of the alveoli. Total pulmonary function is usually recovered during the first year of life but some individuals have permanent deficiency of lung function which affects their exercise tolerance.

Oxygen induced carbon dioxide narcosis occurs in children of any age with chronic respiratory disease, usually cystic fibrosis. Chronic hypoventilation results in retention of carbon dioxide and hypoxia. The respiratory centre adapts to these continuously high levels of carbon dioxide and hypoxia becomes the stimulus to breathe. High concentrations of oxygen given to such children counteracts this hypoxia drive and the child rapidly loses consciousness.

### Incubator

Although the incubator is usually used to provide a constant thermal environment for the neonate, it can also be used as a means of administering oxygen to a concentration of up to 40%. Some incubators have a safety device to prevent the flow of high oxygen concentrations. It is difficult to maintain constant oxygen concentrations as opening of the portholes during nursing causes fluctuations. A perspex head box can be used to reduce these fluctuations.

### Headbox

The headbox is the most efficient way of administering oxygen to an infant. Concentrations of up to 100% can be given in this way. The box is placed over the baby's head taking care that the edges of the box do not rub his neck, chin or shoulders. Anything placed around the edges of the box to prevent rubbing should not prevent the flow of carbon dioxide from the system and the oxygen flow should not be allowed to blow directly into the infant's face. The concentration of the oxygen within the headbox can be monitored by an oxygen analyser. Humidified oxygen should be used wherever possible as it is less irritating to mucous membrane than 'dry' oxygen, but care must be taken to ensure that the nurse's observation of the baby is not obscured by mist.

**Oxygen tent**

For most children over one year of age the oxygen tent is the most efficient method of administering oxygen. Concentrations of up to 40% can be dispersed around the bed or cot with no risk of the oxygen blowing directly into the child's face. It is sometimes difficult to maintain the oxygen concentration and nursing care should be planned carefully to avoid frequent opening of the tent and consequent loss of oxygen. If the tent has been opened for a lengthy period the flow of oxygen should be increased for a few minutes to restore the correct concentration. The enclosed environment can be distressing to some small children who dislike the barrier between them and their mother. This distress can be reduced if a resident parent is close by, but sometimes the child's dyspnoea is so exacerbated by crying that the benefits of using a tent are cancelled out. Humidification is usually used in conjunction with oxygen but the nurse's view of the child should not become obscured by mist on the walls of the tent. The enclosed tent may become very warm but the child's bedding and clothing can become damp from condensation and require frequent changing to avoid chilling. For this reason the temperature within the tent, which should be 6–8 °F lower than room temperature, should be monitored. The child should have some favourite toys with him to minimize fear and boredom but these toys should be washable and not be a fire hazard because of sparks or static electricity.

**Derbyshire chair**

Some of the disadvantages of the oxygen tent can be minimized by the use of the Derbyshire chair. This is an infant chair which has been adapted to include a plastic canopy or hood. This enables a high percentage of oxygen to be given in a relatively enclosed space while the infant remains visible, dry and warm. The upright position also aids respiration by allowing full expansion of the chest. This is probably the optimum method of administering oxygen to infants.

**Face mask**

A face mask is an efficient way of administering oxygen in a range of concentrations up to 100%. It is a suitable method for most school-age children but generally it is best tolerated by older children. A face mask should not be used for children who may vomit and inhale secretions. It has the advantage of allowing easy access to the child. To allow a more comfortable fit, the straps of the mask can be cushioned by foam.

**Nasal catheters and cannulae**

Nasal catheters can provide a high concentration of oxygen continuously. They are inserted nasally to the level of the uvula. In infants nasal catheters occlude most the nasal airway and are thus impractical for use in children of this age group. Older children rarely tolerate the discomfort of this method.

Nasal cannulae are applied just proximal to the opening of the nares. They provide a continuous flow of oxygen and do not interfere with the child's eating and drinking. The only disadvantage of this method is that the oxygen concentration administered is relatively low and cannot be accurately measured.

In most instances of oxygen administration the oxygen supply can be removed while the child is being washed or fed. If necessary, an oxygen source can be held close to the child's face during these activities. During this time the child should be carefully observed for any features which would indicate the need to return to his oxygen supply. Warning features would be a change in colour, increasing respiratory effort or restlessness.

4.2 AEROSOL THERAPY

The purpose of aerosol therapy is to allow the inhalation and deposition of airborne water particles into the respiratory tract. A variety of agents can be used in this way to liquefy secretions, either chemically or by increasing humidity, to reduce oedema of the bronchioles, to dilate swollen and constricted bronchioles or to act against bacterial infection.

There are two main methods of delivering inhaled agents in aerosol form. An aerosol is a colloid system in which solid or liquid particles are suspended in a gas and can be dispensed directly to the respiratory tract in a cloud or mist. A nebulizer is designed to deliver a maximum number of particles of drugs or water to the respiratory tract. They produce an aerosol by forcing oxygen or air through a solution. It takes about 15 min to deliver medication in this way. To simplify and speed up the delivery most drug companies also prepare pressurized aerosols and spinhalers. These containers are small and can be easily carried in the pocket and used anywhere at any time. Figure 4.1 illustrates the different methods of administering aerosol therapy.

The depth of penetration of any medication given by aerosol depends firstly upon the size of the aerosol particles. Most large particles (5–30 $\mu$m) remain trapped in the nose, but the smallest particles (5–0.5 $\mu$m) will reach the alveoli. Pentration and deposition of inhaled particles also depends on the child's breathing pattern. Slow, moderately deep breathing with momentary breath holding at the end of each inspiration will allow optimum delivery of a nebulized solution. Nebulizers can be connected to an oxygen mask for those children who are unable to use the mouthpiece and respond to such instructions. The particles delivered by a pressurized aerosol or spinhaler reach optimum penetration if the aerosol is used after a forced expiration and the drug then inhaled during a deep inspiration. To help children achieve this breathing pattern, some pressurized aerosols and spinhalers are designed to whistle when the correct technique is used.

Studies have shown that medications given by the aerosol method during spontaneous breathing are as effective as those given by intermittent positive pressure ventilator (IPPV) systems. IPPV can cause pneumothorax and airway obstruction by impaction of mucus in the bronchioles in those children who

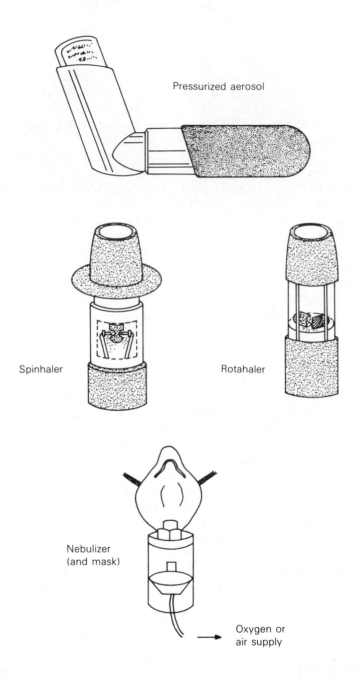

**Figure 4.1** Types of aerosol therapy.

**Table 4.1** Common drugs given by aerosol

| Type and name of drug | Method of inhalation | Action | Side-effects | Precautions |
|---|---|---|---|---|
| *Allergen control*<br>Sodium cromoglycate | Nebulizer, pressurized aerosol or spinhaler | Inhibits the release of chemical mediators, especially histamine in the lung. Must be used regularly for a prophylactic action | Irritation of the throat and trachea by the power resulting in cough or bronchospasm | Decrease dose with care as allergic symptoms may recur |
| *Antibiotics*<br>Gentamycin | Nebulizer | Aminoglycoside which interferes with bacterial protein synthesis | Ototoxicity, nephrotoxicity rashes | Potentiated by diuretics. Can potentiate neuromuscular blocking agents |
| Azlocillin | Nebulizer | Penetrates cell wall of bacteria to interfere with cell wall synthesis | Hypersensitivity, rashes, nausea and diarrhoea | Not to be given to children allergic to penicillin |

**Table 4.1** contd

| Type and name of drug | Method of inhalation | Action | Side-effects | Precautions |
|---|---|---|---|---|
| *Bronchodilators* Ipatropium bromide<br><br>Salbutamol<br><br>Terbutaline | Nebulizer often diluted with normal saline or pressurized aerosol | Causes a 'fear, fright, flight' reaction by stimulating the beta-adrenergic receptors of the autonomic nervous system. This will relax bronchial smooth muscle to cause broncho-dilation. Also results in dilation of coronary vessels, increases the force and rate of cardiac muscle contraction, relaxes alimentary muscles and mobilizes glucose from the liver | Usually due to overdosage or idiosyncratic responses. Stimulation of nervous system – fear, anxiety, tremor, dizziness. Stimulation of cardiovascular system – palpitations, tachycardia, dysrhythmias, hypotension | Not recommended for children under 2 years. Not to be given if child sensitive to atropine. Given with care to child with cardiac disease or hyperthyroidism. Contraindicated for diabetic children. |

| | | | | |
|---|---|---|---|---|
| *Corticosteroids* | | | | |
| Beclomethasone | Nebulizer, pressurized aerosol or spinhaler | Reduction of inflammation aids prophylaxis | Sometimes candidiasis of the mouth and throat. In therapeutic doses should not cause the adverse effects of systemic steroids | Advise children to take a drink following the inhalation of steroids to prevent the drug remaining in the pharyngeal mucosa |
| *Mucolytics* | | | | |
| 0.9% Sodium chloride (normal saline) | Nebulizer (can be used in conjunction with a bronchodilator) | Additional liquid in the respiratory tract reduces the viscosity and tenacity of the sputum | – | – |
| Acetylcysteine | Nebulizer (can be used in conjunction with a bronchodilator) | Ruptures the disulphide bonds of macromolecules which are responsible for the viscosity of mucous secretions. Thus reduces the viscosity and tenacity of sputum, facilitating its removal | Occasionally stomatitis, nausea and vomiting or an irritating cough | Can cause bronchospasm in asthmatic children |

already have high intrapleural pressures. Therefore IPPV should be avoided as a means of giving inhalation therapy to children with asthma or similar conditions.

As with giving any medication, the nurse should familiarize herself with the action, side-effects and special precautions required with drugs given by inhalation. Many medications given in this way are prescribed to be diluted with normal saline to aid the removal of secretions. The effectiveness of any drug is obviously dependent on concentration so the dilution should be accurate. The nurse should educate parents and older children about the drugs to be given so they are aware of expected and undesirable effects (Table 4.1).

### 4.3 PHYSICAL THERAPY

Physical therapy is one of the oldest forms of therapy used to treat disorders of the respiratory tract. It includes chest physiotherapy, which consists of postural drainage, percussion, vibration and coughing, breathing exercises and physical exercises. These are all used both therapeutically and prophylatically to provide mental and physical relaxation, improve posture, strengthen respiratory musculature and improve ventilation. They can be modified to suit the individual needs and abilities of the child. Contraindications to any form of physical therapy are undrained empyema, displaced fractured ribs and excessive pain. Physical therapy is usually performed by the physiotherapist but the nurse should appreciate the technique used and the rationale for each method employed so that she can plan her nursing care appropriately. Physical therapy should be pleasurable to the child if he is to co-operate. The nurse should spend time preparing the child psychologically, and incorporating play into each procedure.

### Chest physiotherapy

The techniques used in chest physiotherapy help to drain and loosen secretions facilitating their removal by expectoration or suction. For those children who have viscous, tenacious sputum, optimum results are obtained if treatment is preceded by a nebulized mucolytic and/or a bronchodilator. The different types of chest physiotherapy are shown in Figure 4.2.

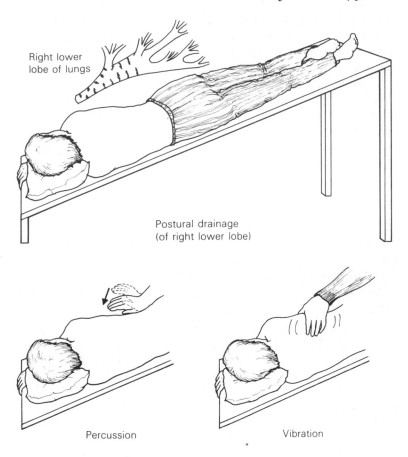

Right lower
lobe of lungs

Postural drainage
(of right lower lobe)

Percussion

Vibration

**Figure 4.2** Types of chest physiotherapy.

## Postural drainage

This method involves placing a specific segmental bronchus in
a vertical position distal to the lung segment which it supplies.
This will allow gravity to assist the downward flow of secretions out of that segement and into larger airways where they
can be more easily removed by coughing or suction. Infants can
be held on the lap of the parent or therapist. Older children can
be positioned on their bed with the end tilted upwards. At
home tilting may be achieved by lying over pillows or over the
side of the bed. Picture books or story books can be placed on
the floor while the child is positioned head downwards.

Postural drainage should be performed 1–1½ h after meals to minimize the possibility of vomiting. The length and duration of the treatment depends on the child's tolerance and physical condition but is usually about 20–30 min. Approximately 5 min is spent in each position. There are nine different positions that can be used to facilitate drainage from each of the main segments of the lung, but usually only five or six positions are used at any one treatment. If a position produces vigorous coughing the child should be allowed to rest before treatment continues.

### Percussion

Percussion – clapping or pummelling – is performed intermittently during postural drainage. It speeds up the drainage of secretions by helping to loosen mucus from the linings of the lower respiratory tract. Vigorous repeated blows are directed at a specific area of the lightly clothed chest wall with cupped hands. A cupped hand creates an air pocket which cushions the blow, and sends a shock wave into the lungs. Performed properly, percussion should make a loud hollow sound and cause no discomfort or pain. A towel, or similar light cloth, should be placed over the area to be treated to prevent stinging. Fingers may have to be used for infants where areas to be percussed may be too small to use the hands.

Children should be reassured that the treatment does not hurt and is not a 'spanking'. They may like to join in the therapy by percussing their teddy bear. Some children find percussion very exhausting and, if this is a severe problem, the procedure may have to be minimal or omitted.

### Vibration

Vibration is a fine shaking motion, performed after postural drainage and percussion, to help move the loosened secretions from the lower airways to the trachea. It is performed only during expiration and the older child is asked to take a deep inhalation and then exhale slowly through pursed lips. Both hands are used to send a vibratory impulse through the chest wall by tensing the muscles of the forearm. Palm or fingers can be used for the smaller child and hand electric vibrators are available for use with premature babies. At the same time as vibrating, pushing up and down on the chest wall will squeeze the underlying structures to further help the movement of secretions. All pressure is released when expiration is completed.

## Coughing and suctioning

Following the above techniques, the older child can be asked to cough and expectorate the secretions which have reached the trachea. The nurse or physiotherapist may have to demonstrate an effective cough – a slow inhalation followed by a forced expiration.

Children who are unable to cough or have suppressed or ineffective coughs must be suctioned. The potential problem of infection and mucosal damage are complications of suctioning adults and children. Suctioning children also has the risks of hypoxia, hypotension and lung collapse. Hypoxia can occur in oxygen dependent children as suction evacuates tracheal gases as well as secretions. Acute hypoxia can cause cardiac arrhythmias. Careful oxygenation and ventilation during the suction procedure should prevent hypoxia. Suction should only be performed for 5 seconds or less as tracheal irritation may cause vagal stimulation and consequent hypotension. It is also important to ensure that suction is carried out with an appropriate size of catheter as too large a catheter will completely occlude small airways. If air cannot enter the lung around the catheter, lung collapse may occur.

### Breathing exercises

Exercises to control breathing (Table 4.2) are beneficial to the child with a chronic respiratory disorder to prevent over-inflation of the lungs, improve the strength of respiratory muscles and increase the effectiveness of the cough. The exercises can incorporate play to make the therapy into a game. Children can be taught to participate in breathing exercises from about three years old.

### Physical exercise

Moderate exercise is usually advantageous for children with chronic respiratory disorders. Activities which do not overtax

**Table 4.2** Techniques to improve breathing

| Technique | Purpose | Instructions | Use of play |
|---|---|---|---|
| Pursed lip breathing | To prevent over-inflation | Purse lips, inhale slowly through the nose and then slowly exhale | Whistling; blowing bubbles |
| Abdominal or diaphragmatic breathing | To improve the strength of the abdominal muscles and aid respiration | Inhale through the nose with a relaxed abdomen. Inhale through pursed lips while a helper pushes inwards and upwards to help the diaphragm move upwards. During exhalation use the abdominal muscles to help to force out air | Blowing a small ball along a table. Blowing bubbles. A teddy bear on the abdomen will fall over as the abdominal muscle contracts |
| Expansion of the lower chest | To maintain good movement of the lower chest | Place the palm of the hand over the lower ribs and apply gentle pressure. During inspiration try to move the lower ribs against the hand. Release the pressure during exhalation | – |
| Forced expiration 'huffing' | To improve the efficiency of coughing and expectoration | Take a medium breath in and then give a forced and slightly prolonged breath out | Paper windmill |

the respiratory system, but need controlled rates of breathing, help to maximize respiratory function and maintain posture. Running, tennis, cricket and swimming are all useful sports which should be encouraged within the individual child's inclination, ability and aptitude. Those children who do not do any physical exercise should be taught good posture to prevent the development of round shoulders.

Stretching exercises increase the flexibility of the intercostal muscles. Sit-ups and leg raising exercises help to strengthen the abdominal muscles to improve the quality of expiration.

# 5 Care of the neonate with respiratory distress syndrome

Respiratory distress in the newborn baby can be seen as a result of hypovolaemia, hypoglycaemia, congenital heart disease and cerebral haemorrhage. However, the term 'respiratory distress syndrome' is applied to a condition which is associated with the immature lungs of the preterm infant. It is also sometimes seen in babies of diabetic mothers and those born by caesarian section. Although improved methods of treatment in the last 20 years have reduced the number of deaths, respiratory distress syndrome still has a high mortality and morbidity rate. Advances in mechanical ventilation, techniques for predicting fetal lung maturity and the administration of glucocorticoids antenatally to improve lung maturity at birth have all helped to keep more babies alive. However, the babies who survive have a high risk of developing long-term complications such as intraventricular haemorrhage. Respiratory distress syndrome (RDS) may also be known as 'idiopathic respiratory distress syndrome' (IRDS) or 'hyaline membrane disease' (HMD).

## 5.1 PATHOPHYSIOLOGY

The infant born at term can adapt relatively easily to the respiratory changes necessary to enable the lungs to take over responsibility for gaseous exchange. The lungs of the premature infant are too immature to cope with these essential alterations. The alveoli of the preterm infant are much smaller in diameter (75 $\mu$m) than those of the full-term infant (100 $\mu$m). These tiny alveoli are difficult to inflate and, once inflated, it is difficult to maintain the inflation. One of the reasons for this is the lack of surfactant. Acting like a detergent, surfactant is secreted by mature aleveolar epithelium to reduce the surface tension of fluids in the lining of the respiratory system. Without surfactant there is a high surface tension, especially at the end of expiration, which causes alveolar collapse and atelectasis. The force necessary to maintain alveolar patency is explained by Laplace's law:

$$P \text{ (distending pressure)} = \frac{2 \times \text{surface tension}}{r \text{ (alveolar radius)}}$$

The premature infant who has immature lungs has a small alveolar radius and a high surface tension. Both of these factors require a high intra-alveolar pressure to maintain alveolar inflation. A high intrathoracic pressure can be produced by deep inspirations but the premature baby lacks the necessary muscle and strength in his chest wall to be able to do this. In addition, the abnormally elastic ribs of the preterm infant increase the pliability of the chest wall causing it to partially collapse with each contraction of the diaphragm. The low intrathoracic pressure and increased flexibility of the thoracic cavity both aggravate atelectasis.

Widespread atelectasis causes hypoxia and hypercapnia. Prolonged hypoxia activates anaerobic glycolysis which produces an increased amount of lactic acid. Increased lactic acid causes a metabolic acidosis but the collapsed lungs do not have the ability to compensate for this by blowing off excess carbon dioxide. Thus, a respiratory acidosis is produced. The decrease in pH causes vasoconstriction, impairing the pulmonary circulation. This produces a vicious circle of a deficient pulmonary circulation and alveolar perfusion causing a fall in $pO_2$ and pH. It also means that materials needed for the production of surfactant cannot be circulated to the alveoli. Instead, hypoxia and increased pulmonary vascular pressure cause transudation of fluid from the pulmonary vessels into the alveoli to form a hyaline membrane. This membrane causes further difficulties with respiration as it decreases the elasticity of the lung tissue. The affected lungs are more rigid and require even more pressure to achieve inflation.

## 5.2 CLINICAL FEATURES

Babies with respiratory distress syndrome develop progressive respiratory insufficiency which begins either at birth or within a few hours afterwards. The affected infant may at first appear to breathe normally and be a healthy pink colour, but within 30 min to 2 h after birth, he gradually becomes more dyspnoeic and substernal retractions may be seen.

Soon afterwards this respiratory distress becomes more obvious. Breathing is more laboured, the rate of respiration may increase up to 80–120 breaths/min and the substernal retractions become more prominent. To endeavour to overcome the collapse of the alveoli the glottis partially closes at the end of expiration to increase airway pressure. This is shown by an audible expiratory grunt. Flaring of the external nares and cyanosis accompanies these signs of severe respiratory distress. The increased work of respiration together with hypoxia causes fatigue and the affected infant gradually becomes more flaccid, inert and unresponsive.

## 5.3 INVESTIGATIONS

Chest X-ray shows a typical picture of a diffuse granular pattern due to the small, closely spaced density representing the areas of collapse.

Arterial blood gas tensions and pH will reveal a $pO_2$ of less than 50 mmHg, a $pCO_2$ of greater than 50 mmHg and a pH of less than 7.3. Arterial samples are collected at least every 2–4 h to monitor the course of the condition. They can be taken from an umbilical artery catheter or drawn off by needle puncture to the radial, pedal or temporal arteries. To avoid repeated punctures percutaneous blood gas analysis may be used. Table 5.1 shows normal arterial blood valves.

**Table 5.1** Arterial blood values relating to pulmonary function

| Determination | Premature infant | Newborn | | | Child |
|---|---|---|---|---|---|
| | | *1–4 h* | *12–24 h* | *24–28 h* | |
| $pO_2$ mmHg | 60 | 62 | 68 | 63–87 | 100 |
| $pCO_2$ mmHg | 40 | 39 | 33 | 34 | 35–45 |
| pH | 7.35 | 7.3 | 7.39 | 7.39 | 7.38–7.42 |

## 5.4 MEDICAL MANAGEMENT

With medical intervention respiratory distress syndrome is self-limiting. Although the infant deteriorates rapidly at first and continues to do so for the initial 48 h after birth, improvement usually occurs by 72 h as surfactant production increases. Thus, the management of the syndrome is mostly supportive and includes all the general measures required by any preterm infant. Unfortunately, the complications of the disease itself and the treatment are numerous and can prolong the course of events. Pulmonary ischaemia, high pulmonary oxygen concentrations and positive pressure ventilation can cause further damage to the respiratory system and chronic lung disease. Positive pressure ventilation can cause rupture of the alveoli and, as a consequence, air leaks into the pleural cavity, mediastinum, pericardium or peritoneum. Other complications include patent ductus arteriosus and heart failure, intraventricular haemorrhage, secondary infection and multiple metabolic problems.

The specific aims of management are to correct acidosis, to maintain a neutral thermal environment and conserve utilization of oxygen, and to provide additional inspired oxygen. Respiratory acidosis is treated by correcting the contributing factors: stress, hypoglycaemia and hypocalaemia. Intravenous dextrose (10%) via a peripheral line can be given to maintain a blood glucose of 2–4 mmol/l. This will also provide nutritional intake for the firt 48 h when feeding via the gastrointestinal tract is impossible. The preterm baby often has physical difficulty in sucking and swallowing, digesting and absorbing his feed, so when feeds commence on the third day of life or when the baby's condition is more stable, they are given by the nasojejunal route. Small feeds (2–3 ml/kg) are given at intervals of 2–3 h.

Parenteral fluids are commenced at 60–80 ml/kg 24 h to avoid over-infusion, pulmonary oedema and the development of heart failure. Hypovolaemia must also be avoided as the resulting hypotension will aggravate pulmonary ischaemia. An optimum fluid intake should produce an urinary output of 2 ml/kg/h with a specific gravity of less than 1.01. The serum calcium level can be maintained by the addition of calcium gluconate 200 mg/kg/24 h. Potassium and chloride are not usually given until the second day of life.

**Table 5.2** Common methods of assisted ventilation in respiratory distress syndrome

| Method | Description | Criteria | Provision | Precautions |
|---|---|---|---|---|
| Supplemental oxygen | 60% to 80% oxygen | If $pO_2$ = 50–70 mmHg | Head box | |
| Continuous positive airway pressure (CPAP) | Provides constant distending pressure to the airway of an infant who is breathing spontaneously | If $pO_2$ > 50 mmHg | Nasotracheal intubation | Pressures over 10 cm $H_2O$ may cause pulmonary air leaks. As infant improves decrease CPAP slowly or massive atelectasis may occur |
| Positive end-expiratory presure (PEEP) | Provides an increased transpulmonary pressure at the end of expiration to prevent alveolar collapse | If $pO_2$ > 50 mmHg with 100% oxygen and CPAP of 10 cm $H_2O$ or infant is apnoeic on CPAP or $pO_2$ < 50 mmHg | Nasotracheal intubation | Use lowest pressures to avoid the development of bronchopulmonary dysplasia |

Additional inspired oxygen is provided by increasing the ambient oxygen contraction or by assisted ventilation. Oxygen therapy in this situation aims to overcome hypoxia, prevent the accumulation of lactic acid and avoid the toxic effects of oxygen in the preterm infant. The method of improving oxygenation is dependent on the infant's blood gases but the most commonly used method is mechanical ventilation (Table 5.2). As the infant improves any respiratory support should be withdrawn gradually to prevent relapse. He will usually require supplemental oxygen for several days after extubation, when he is still in the recovery phase.

## 5.5 NURSING CARE

Care of the infant with respiratory distress syndrome will include all the nursing care necessary for a premature baby. In addition, particular care and attention is required to maintain the infant's airway and adequate ventilation. The infant will be admitted soon after birth so mother will not be available. The birth of a premature baby is usually unexpected and a frightening event for both parents and the removal of the baby to a special unit adds to their fears and uncertainty. They need support and explanations to help them come to terms with the situation. Separation of mother and baby may severely affect the bonding process. A mother demonstrates a predictable and orderly pattern of behaviour during the development of the attachment bond with her baby during the first few days of his life. Physical separation of mother and baby soon after birth prevents this emotional relationship from occurring and can seriously damage the mother's ability for mothering her child. A polaroid photograph of the baby can be taken to enable the mother to have some link with him until she is discharged.

Recent studies have also shown how stressful a neonatal intensive care unit can be for the infant. Sound levels and the intensity of continuous light are higher than in a ward situation. It is important, however, to ensure that the infant receives the tactile, visual and auditory stimuli that the healthy neonate would receive.

### Assessment

A premature baby with respiratory distress syndrome will be

admitted as an emergency. The nurse will have little time on admission to assess the infant but while she is settling him she can make a quick assessment of the more pertinent details which will allow her to plan her initial care.

### Breathing and circulation

- What is the baby's heart and respiratory rate?
- Does he show any signs of respiratory distress?

### Maintaining normal body temperature

- Is the baby hypothermic?

### Elimination

- Is there abdominal distension which may further embarrass respiratory function?

### Communication

- Where will the parents be based? How can they be contacted?
- Has a photograph of the baby been taken to be given to the mother?
- What do they know about their baby's condition?
- What name has been given to the baby?

### Mobilizing

- How does the baby respond to handling?

### Dying

- Do the parents want their baby christened?
- What is the baby's weight? (The weight of the infant correlates with the incidence of perinatal mortality and morbidity.)

**Planning**

A neutral thermal environment helps to prevent cold stress due to excessive heat loss and conserves oxygen. The baby should be nursed in an incubator to maintain his temperature at 36.5–37.2°C. All care must be carefully planned to avoid overhandling of the infant and frequent opening of the incubator portholes as this will quickly cause the baby's temperature to fall. His extremities should be kept covered to minimize heat loss. A daily record of the baby's weight should be kept; if he is using all his metabolic energy to keep warm he may not be able to gain weight.

The next most essential aspect of nursing care is the continuous assessment of the infant's condition to assess his response to therapy and help the early detection of complications. Close observation of the baby's colour, chest movements and respiratory effort should be made. He should be positioned on his side or prone to allow easy drainage of mucus. In the early stages of respiratory distress syndrome secretions are minimal but following intubation excessive thick tenacious secretions are produced which interfere with gas flow and predispose to asphyxia. Suctioning may be required two hourly and the quantity and character or oral, pharyngeal and tracheal secretions should be recorded. Chest physiotherapy is essential to aid in the removal of secretions and prevent atelectasis and pneumonia, and the nurse should liaise with the physiotherapist so that their care is coordinated.

Once the infant's mother is discharged from the maternity ward care should also be planned to include her. She should be encouraged to visit as soon and as much as possible. She should be helped to become actively involved in her baby's care and allowed to hold and cuddle him as much as possible. The nurse should be available to give support especially at the first visit but she should also recognize that the new mother needs time alone with her baby to develop a relationship with him. The nurse should also be aware that both parents may become tense with anxiety and tiredness and she may need to suggest rest periods away from the unit.

Table 5.3 illustrates a nursing care plan for a typical case of a premature baby with respiratory distress syndrome.

## 5.6 HEALTH EDUCATION

The most successful approach to the prevention of deaths and handicaps resulting from respiratory distress syndrome is the

**Table 5.3** Care of the premature baby with respiratory distress syndrome. David Birch was born at 25 weeks gestation, arriving by spontaneous vaginal delivery. His birth weight was 900 g. His Apgar scores were 3 at 1 min, 6 at 5 min and 8 at 10 min. He was immediately transferred to the special care baby unit, intubated and given continuous positive airway pressure ventilation. An intravenous infusion of 10% dextrose was commenced to give him 100 ml/kg/day. A chest X-ray showed the presence of hyaline membrane disease and it was decided to transfer David to the regional neonatal centre. On arrival, David's colour was pink and he had good chest expansion. His father, who was extremely anxious about the condition of his first child, accompanied him but planned to return to his wife as soon as possible

| Problem | Aim of care | Nursing intervention |
|---------|-------------|----------------------|
| Potential respiratory distress due to immature lungs and/or adverse effects of mechanical ventilation | To ensure David's spontaneous breathing is supported effectively at 40–60 breaths/min | Continuous positive airway pressure ventilation with a pressure of 8 cm $H_2O$ and using 100% oxygen<br>Note chest movements, colour and character of breath sounds hourly for any signs of distress |
| Potential airway obstruction due to excess secretions | To promote free drainage of secretions | Position David prone or on either side<br>Record the quantity and character of secretions<br>Suction nasotracheal tube at least 2 hourly after insertion of 0.3–0.5 ml normal saline<br>Chest physiotherapy at least 4 hourly<br>Keep humidifier filled with sterile water |
| Potential hypoxia due to failure of the ventilator | To ensure continuous ventilation is maintained | Prevent kinking or displacement of ventilator tubing<br>Move child carefully and slowly and leave enough slack in tubing to prevent accidental disconnection |

| Problem | Goal | Nursing action |
|---|---|---|
| Potential complications of oxygen therapy (brain damage due to hypoxia, lung and/or eye damage from hyperoxia) | (a) To ensure David's pO$_2$ remains between 50 and 70 mmHg<br>(b) To monitor David for signs of complications | Apply transcutaneous oxygen monitor, changing electrodes 4 hourly<br>Report any fluctuations shown on monitor<br>Observe fontanelles for tenseness or bulging |
| Potential increased metabolic rate and oxygen consumption due to heat loss | To maintain David's body temperature 36.5–37.2°C | Nurse in incubator at 32–35°C<br>Attach temperature probe and observe monitor hourly<br>Dress in hat and bootees and cover with warmed Gamgee<br>Plan care to avoid frequent handling and opening portholes<br>Weigh daily to monitor metabolic rate |
| Potential hypoglycaemia due to reduced glycogen storage | To maintain David's Dextrostix at 2.0–4.0 mmol/l | IVI dextrose 10% 3 ml/h<br>2 hourly Dextrostix |
| Potential worsening of respiratory status due to fluid and electrolyte imbalance | To maintain David's urine output at 2 ml/h with a specific gravity of no more than 1.010 | Measure urine output hourly<br>Test all urine for specific gravity<br>Record all intake and output<br>Observe for signs of electrolye imbalance (lethargy, hyperactivity, twitching) |

Check ventilator settings hourly
Check that hand ventilation equipment is functioning daily
Check all ventilator connections are secure

**Table 5.3** contd

| Problem | Aim of care | Nursing intervention |
| --- | --- | --- |
| Potential infection due to immature immune system | (a) To maintain protective precautions<br>(b) To keep David's skin and mucous membranes in healthy condition | Wash and dry hands before handling David<br>Allow only parents and grandparents to visit<br>Keep skin clean and dry<br>Give mouth care 2 hourly<br>Observe eyes, umbilical area and infusion site for any inflammation |
| Potential exhaustion due to lack of energy reserves | To ensure David's heart rate remains within normal limits (100–140/min) | Plan care to provide maximal rest time between procedures<br>Avoid cold stress (see above)<br>Record pulse 2 hourly |
| David and his mother have been separated | To enable Mrs Birch to keep in touch | Take a polaroid picture of David for Mr Birch to take to his wife<br>Arrange way of informing Mrs Birch of David's progress |
| Parental anxiety | To help David's father to feel more relaxed and to understand David's condition | Explain ward layout and routine<br>Describe and explain all nursing care and treatment |
| Potential disturbance in David's development due to lack of appropriate stimulation | To provide appropriate sensory stimulation | Talk to David during care<br>Provide skin contact when caring for David and hold your face within 9–12 inches of him<br>Put mobiles in field of vision<br>Avoid loud noises and bright lights |

prevention of premature births. More attention may need to be given to preconceptual health education to ensure an optimum environment for the developing fetus.

Amniocentesis can determine fetal lung maturity by assessing the amniotic fluid lecithin/sphingomyelin ratio. This allows a reasonable prediction of whether a fetus is likely to develop respiratory distress syndrome and may be useful when an elective early delivery is being considered.

Corticosteroids, administered to pregnant mothers for 1–7 days prior to an early delivery, appear to stimulate the production of surfactant and reduce the incidence of respiratory distress syndrome.

Recent research is based on surfactant replacement therapy. Exogenous surfactant has been administered intratracheally to preterm infants in clinical trials. These infants have shown significantly improved gaseous exchange and require less oxygen and mechanical ventilation. However, a number of points still needs clarification. The exact dose and frequency is unsure and it is also not known how this replacement therapy affects the body's own ability to synthesize endogenous surfactant.

# 6 Care of the young infant with bronchiolitis

Bronchiolitis is one of the more common infectious diseases of the lower respiratory tract characterized by severe mechanical and inflammatory changes in the bronchioles. Acute infections involving the respiratory tract are the most common types of illness in young children. Infants and pre-school children usually have four or five such infections each year, varying in severity from mild to life threatening. The severity of these illnesses and the child's response to the infection is related to several factors:

- The nature of the infecting agent.
- The degree and frequency of the exposure to the infection.
- The age of the child (infants have less resistance to infection and their smaller airways are subject to severe narrowing from inflammation).
- General health of the child. (Malnutrition, anaemia and immune deficiency disorders increase the likelihood of infection.)
- Other disorders of the respiratory tract. (The presence of other respiratory disorders such as allergies or cystic fibrosis weaken respiratory defence mechanisms.)

## 6.1 AETIOLOGY

### Incidence

Bronchiolitis usually occurs in children between the ages of 2 and 12 months with a peak incidence at 6 months. Infant mortality figures show bronchiolitis as the number three cause of death. It can occur in young children up to the age of 2 years but it is rare after this time. There is an increased incidence in those infants who were born prematurely due to both their immature respiratory system and their lack of immunity. It is more common in males than females.

Bronchiolitis occurs more often in the winter and spring months, usually as a result of an upper respiratory tract infection.

## Causative organisms

Bronchiolitis is mainly a viral illness caused predominantly by the respiratory syncytial virus. This particular virus, which has been a suspected cause of sudden infant death syndrome, is a specific virus isolated from children with an infection involving the airways of the lower respiratory tract. It is named from its ability to cause syncytium formation (a multinucleate mass of protoplasm produced by the merging of cells) in tissue culture. Adenoviruses, parainfluenza and influenza viruses can also cause viral bronchiolitis. Mycoplasma pneumonia, an aerobic, gram-negative microorganism without a cell wall, classified between bacteria and viruses, is a less common cause of bronchiolitis.

## Transmission

The respiratory tract is lined with mucous membrane throughout and, as a result, respiratory tract infections are rarely confined to one structure but tend to spread to nearby areas within the respiratory system. Bronchiolitis usually begins as a minor upper respiratory tract infection which is spread by inhalation. The causative organisms are suspended in the air by talking, coughing or sneezing. They can remain airborne and infectious for an hour or more to be inhaled by others. As discussed above, infants and young children are more susceptible to such organisms.

## 6.2 PATHOPHYSIOLOGY

Respiratory viruses primarily attack the epithelial cells of the upper respiratory tract, causing inflammation and desquamation. As the organisms multiply large numbers of cilia are

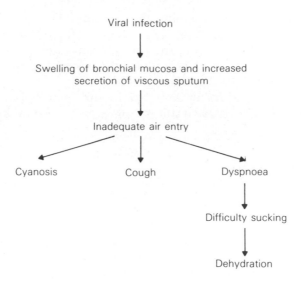

**Figure 6.1**  The progression of bronchiolitis.

destroyed. The cilia and mucus normally form a protective layer to trap foreign particles and transport them along the tracheo-bronchial tree for expectoration or swallowing. When this line of defence is impaired the organisms are able to continue multiplying and to reach the bronchi and bronchioles. The epithelial cells of these structures are then infiltrated causing interstitial inflammation and desquamation. The mucosa of the bronchioles swells and the lumen fills with mucus and exudate. The small airways of the infants may be severely obstructed by such changes. This narrowing impairs ventilation by trapping air in the airways above the obstructed areas. The trapped air hinders the normal exchange of gases and hyperinflation occurs in an effort to compensate for this. As a result dilation of the bronchioles occurs. When inspired air reaches the dilated area the pressure is reduced, in turn there is a decrease in alveolar air pressure and a further reduction in adequate ventilation. Air is also trapped distal to the obstructed areas. This air diffuses into the pulmonary circulation but cannot be replaced with fresh inspired air. As a result the alveoli in the affected area shrink and collapse.

Bronchiolitis may cause further problems in the small child. The smaller airways can become totally obstructed causing apnoeic attacks. The small child becomes easily exhausted from the effort to take in oxygen and anoxia and circulatory collapse may ensue. The immature immunity of the small child together with his inability to expectorate mucus and exudate enables secondary bacterial infection to occur (Figure 6.1).

## 6.3 CLINICAL FEATURES

The onset of bronchiolitis is usually gradual, beginning insiduously with a simple upper respiratory infection. The child has a serous nasal discharge accompanied by a low grade pyrexia. After 48–72 h he becomes more distressed. Increased respiratory distress is shown by dyspnoea, tachypnoea, with flaring nares and subcostal and intercostal retractions. Coarse rattling sounds can be heard during expiration and the fever becomes more pronounced. There may also be wheezing and cyanosis if there is widespread obstruction of the airways.

Infants and young children tend to react more severely to acute respiratory infections than older children and adults. They usually demonstrate generalized features as well as localized signs and symptoms relating to the respiratory tract. An infant or small child with bronchiolitis may therefore also present with any or all of the following:

- *Cough*. The infant over the age of 6 months may have a dry cough.
- *Nasal blockage*. Infants have small nasal passages which are easily blocked by mucus and exudate. As a consequence their main means of air entry is impaired.
- *Pyrexia*. Children under 5 years have difficult maintaining their body temperature especially in the presence of infection.
- *Febrile convulsions*. In severe infections a sudden rise in body temperature to 40°C or above may cause a brief, generalized convulsion.
- *Poor feeding patterns*. Anorexia commonly accompanies most acute infections in children. In respiratory infections the problem is compounded by the need to breathe through the mouth.
- *Diarrhoea and vomiting*. Viral infections in small children are commonly accompanied by some gastrointestinal disturbance. If severe the child may also show features of dehydration.

- *Abdominal pain.* Small children with acute respiratory infection complain of abdominal pain often due to abdominal distension. This distension further hampers breathing.

## 6.4 INVESTIGATIONS

The clinical features, as described above, are fairly non specific but a chest X-ray will help in determining the diagnosis of bronchiolitis by showing overinfiltration of the lungs. If necessary, a throat swab will isolate the causative organism by virological or serological tests. Blood gases will reveal a decreased $pO_2$.

## 6.5 MEDICAL MANAGEMENT

Hospitalization is usually desirable for the infant with bronchiolitis. Although the infection is usually of short duration (7–10 days) and has a good prognosis, the young infant usually requires alternative methods of feeding during the acute phase to prevent dehydration and fluid and electrolyte imbalance. He also requires careful monitoring to note signs of respiratory acidosis, apnoeic spells or circulatory collapse. Humidified oxygen helps to relieve hypoxia but blood gases must be checked daily initially to ensure acid/base balance. Ventilatory support is sometimes required to correct acidosis.

The management is mainly conservative. Antiobiotics are not usually given as the causative organism is commonly a virus. Bronchodilators are not indicated as bronchospasm does not occur and corticosteroids have not proved effective. Cough suppressants or expectorants for the dry cough are not appropriate for the small children affected by bronchiolitis who are largely unable to cough or expectorate properly. Sedation for any respiratory disorder is unadvisable as it will depress the laboured respiratory rate even further.

## 6.6 NURSING CARE

**Assessment**

*Breathing*

- What is the child's respiratory rate and pattern?
- Is there any nasal flaring and/or abnormal chest movements?

- What is the child's colour?
- Is there any wheezing or other breath sounds?
- Has he any nasal obstruction?
- Has he got a cough? What does the cough sound like?

*Maintaining body temperature*

- What is the child's temperature?

*Eating and drinking*

- Is the child taking feeds as usual?

*Elimination*

- Has there been any associated vomiting or diarrhoea?

*Rest and sleep*

- Does he appear restless, lethargic or exhaused?

*Communication*

- Has the child complained of, or appeared to suffer from any pain?
- Has he become quieter or more irritable with the course of the infection?

*Maintaining a safe environment*

- Does the child show any signs of dehydration (tachycardia, hypotension, dry inelastic skin, sunken eyes and fontanelle)?

**Planning**

The child requires an atmosphere of high humidity to loosen the mucus and exudate present in the bronchioles and supplemental oxygen to relieve dyspnoea and hypoxia. The exact position of the child will vary according to his age. Infants of 3 months or less are usually nursed in a headbox with the head of the cot tilted upwards. Older babies can be positioned in a baby seat inside an oxygen tent. Infants should be given nasopharyngeal suction as necessary to clear nasal mucus and help

**Table 6.1** Care of the infant with bronchiolitis. Jane Elliot, aged 3 months, has been admitted with bronchiolitis. She became ill with a runny nose and slight temperature 2 days previously. On admission, she is breathing with difficulty, her respiratory rate is 60/min and she shows signs of nasal flaring and intercostal retractions. She is weak but irritable. Her mother reports that she has not been taking her breast feeds well and has had some vomiting and diarrhoea. Mother plans to visit during the day when Jane's brothers are at school

| Problem | Aim of care | Nursing intervention |
| --- | --- | --- |
| Potential blockage of airway by secretions | Jane's airway will remain clear | Tilt head of cot up<br>Nasopharyngeal suction to clear nasal secretions<br>Nurse on apnoea mattress<br>Chest physiotherapy three times daily |
| Respiratory distress | Jane will be able to breathe more easily at a rate of 35–45/min | Nurse in headbox with 40% humidified oxygen<br>Record respirations 2 hourly<br>Report increased dyspnoea, cyanosis and continued nasal flaring and chest retractions |
| Pyrexia | Jane's temperature will be within normal limits | Provide cool environment and clothing<br>Administer Calpol as prescribed when temperature 38°C or above<br>Record temperature hourly while pyrexial |
| Potential secondary infection due to immature immunity | Jane will not develop any further infection while in hospital | Nurse in a cubicle with protective precautions<br>Observe secretions for signs of further infection (purulent, thicker) |

| Potential dehydration due to difficulty with feeding | Jane will remain hydrated and have an intake of at least 800 ml/24 h | Maintain intravenous fluids at the prescribed rate<br>Offer 5–10 ml clear fluid as desired when less breathless<br>Record all intake and output<br>Weigh daily<br>Record urinary specific gravity<br>Note any features of dehydration (dry skin, sunken fontanelle, oliguria, concentrated urine, weight loss) |
| Potential circulatory collapse due to exhaustion | Jane will have sufficient physical and psychological rest to maintain a pulse rate of 100–140 beats/min | Plan care to promote rest<br>Anticipate Jane's needs<br>Record pulse rate hourly – report any deviations |
| Potential excoriation of buttocks from diarrhoea | Jane's napkin area will remain clean, dry and healthy | Change nappy as soon as soiling occurs<br>Apply barrier cream to napkin area |
| Parental anxiety and apprehension | Mr and Mrs Elliot will be less fearful about Jane's care | Include parents in Jane's care<br>Allay any guilt about not being resident<br>Explain all nursing intervention<br>Follow Mrs Elliot's normal routine for Jane's care wherever possible |

to maintain a clear airway as infants breathe through their noses. Dyspnoea and the exhaustion this produces usually makes it difficult for the infant to take his usual feed. There is also a danger of aspiration of feed if the infant is in severe respiratory distress. As babies are nose breathers, intragastric feeding via nasogastric or nasojejunal tube is not always appropriate. Intravenous fluids are usually the method of choice to allow the child to rest and also to maintain his nutrition and fluid and electrolyte balance. The infant should be weighed daily and an accurate fluid chart maintained to evaluate these aspects. Table 6.1 illustrates the typical care plan of a child with bronchiolitis.

Vital signs should be recorded at least 4 hourly to enable the nurse to be alert for signs of complications. Increased difficulty in breathing, cyanosis, tachycardia weakness are all indications of deterioration. An apnoea mattress should be used to give immediate warning of any apnoeic spells.

As the infant's breathing becomes less distressed, the oxygen concentration can be decreased and small amounts of clear fluid offered orally. If these are tolerated with no change in colour, respiratory and pulse rate, the oxygen can gradually be discontinued and normal feeds recommenced. As the child begins to take more by mouth the intravenous rate can be adjusted to prevent fluid overload. Once a normal feed pattern is re-established the intravenous fluids can also be discontinued.

## 6.7 HEALTH EDUCATION

Parents of young children should be aware of the infant's lowered resistance to respiratory tract infections. Within reason they should try to avoid bringing their infant into contact with those who have a respiratory infection or taking him to crowded places where such infections are easily transmitted. They should accept that young children ordinarily have several acute respiratory infections each year, the majority of which may be quite trivial, but they should also know when to seek medical advice. Any degree of respiratory distress, pallor or blueness of the lips, restlessness and high temperature should be reported to the general practitioner. Parents who smoke should also realize that cigarette smoke in the atmosphere compromises the infant's natural defence mechanisms further by depressing ciliary action and can make him even more susceptible to respiratory tract infections.

# 7 Care of the infant with whooping cough

Whooping cough, or pertussis, is a bacterial disease which is highly infectious. The infection primarily affects the respiratory system, resulting in paroxysmal coughing and sudden forceful inspirations. These sudden inspirations give a high-pitched crowing sound or 'whoop' which gives the disease its common name.

Whooping cough is a potentially serious disease and can be fatal. In 1982, there were 14 deaths from whooping cough in England and Wales. Approximately 10% of children develop the disease so severely that hospital admission is neccesary. In infants under 6 months this figure increases to 60%. There is also evidence to show that severe whooping cough has long-term consequences (Johnson et al., 1985). Children who have been admitted to hospital with severe whooping cough do not perform as well in educational tests at the age of 5 years. Chronic respiratory problems, such as bronchiectasis, may also be a result on whooping cough.

## 7.1 AETIOLOGY

### Incidence

Whooping cough can occur at any age but is more commonly seen in children under 5 years of age. The greatest mortality and morbidity occurs in babies under 1 year, especially females. Whooping cough occurs throughout the year although there is sometimes a slight increase in the number of cases in the summer months. It also tends to occur more frequently every 3 to 4 years. It occurs throughout the world but its incidence

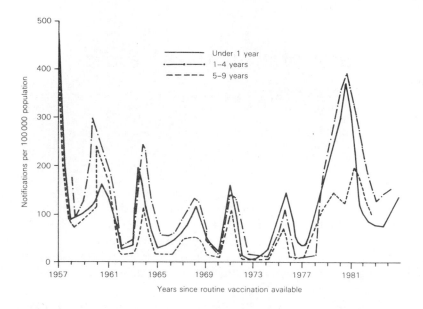

**Figure 7.1** Notifications of whooping cough.

and effect vary. This difference is caused by social, economic, political and physical factors. Whooping cough is more prevalent in densely populated big cities. In 1941, one of the largest epidemics of the disease occurred when city children, evacuated to the country during the bombing of the large cities, transmitted the disease to the children of the more sparsely populated areas who, until this time, had been largely unaffected.

Health care facilities in different parts of the world also affect the incidence of the condition. The availability and effectiveness of an immunization programme causes a variation in the incidence of whooping cough. Whooping cough vaccine was introduced in this country in 1942. Although it was available in some local authorities from this time it did not become available nationally until 1957. In 1956 about 1300/100 000 individuals contracted the disease. This figure dropped to 500/100 000 the following year with the nationwide introduction of the vaccine, and continued to decrease until 1978. In

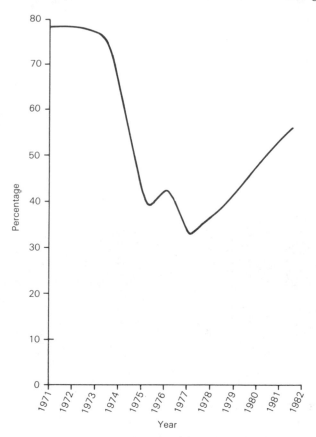

**Figure 7.2** Percentage of the infant population vaccinated against whooping cough.

1974, adverse publicity about the side-effects of the vaccine caused such concern about the efficacy of immunization that the uptake of vaccination fell to only 37% and the incidence of whooping cough in 1978, the next 4-yearly peak, increased to 900/100 000 (Figure 7.1). In 1985, the World Health Organization reported a decrease in the notified cases of whooping cough presumably due to more widespread vaccination. For instance, North Africa had a lower incidence of the disease although only half their children had been vaccinated. The number of deaths from whooping cough also varies with the standard of health care. The quality of health care facilities, the availability of drugs such as antibiotics and an effective

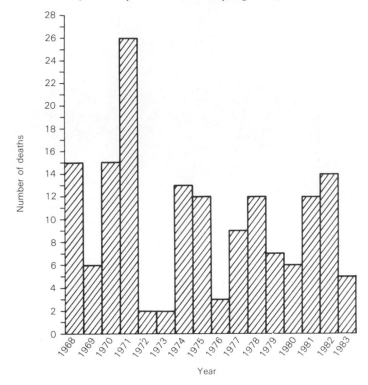

**Figure 7.3**  Deaths from whooping cough.

immunization programme can all alter the death rate. In 1983, the World Health Organisation reported that New Zealand, with a population of three million, had had no deaths from whooping cough. In contrast to this, Guatemala, with a population of six million, had 1102 deaths. The death rate from whooping cough in the UK fell dramatically in the 1950s following the introduction of antibiotics for the treatment of pneumonia, the commonest cause of death from whooping cough. Between 1977 and 1978 when the uptake of vaccination fell by 43%, the death rate in England and Wales rose from three in 1976 to 27 (Figures 7.2 and 7.3).

### Causative organism

The causative organism of whooping cough is a bacteria, *Bordetella pertussis*, but it is known that related organisms such as *B. parapertussis* and *B. bronchoseptica* and some adenoviruses can also cause clinical features of whooping cough.

### Transmission

Whooping cough is highly infectious. The infection is transmitted by droplet infection from person to person. The incubation period is variable but it is usually 7–10 days. If an individual has not developed the clinical features of the disease 14 days after coming into contact with the disease, he will not develop it. The period of infectivity lasts for 4 weeks after the onset of symptoms, the first 2 weeks being the time of highest risk.

The under-5s are most at risk from developing the infection. Epidemics can readily occur in nursery schools where some vaccinated children are exposed to such large doses of bacteria from their infected classmates that they too contract the infection. Children under 5 can readily infect their younger siblings, especially those too young for vaccination. They may also infect their parents. The few incidents of adults who have contracted whooping cough for the second time are mostly parents, especially mothers. Immunity following a natural infection with *B. pertussis* is lifelong, but older children and adults who have not had natural whooping cough may not be protected by the immunization they received during infancy. As the worldwide incidence of whooping cough decreases, and therefore the number of individuals with natural immunity, it is essential to isolate individuals for at least 2 weeks after the onset of features.

### 7.2 PATHOPHYSIOLOGY

Initially, the presence of *B. pertussis* in the upper respiratory tract causes an inflammatory reaction of the mucous membranes of the nose, throat and bronchi. The bacteria adhere to the ciliated epithelial lining of these structures inhibiting its function, and cellular debris, mucus and pus collect. In some areas this waste material causes plugging of the bronchial tree resulting in necrosis of the bronchial epithelium. The lung tissue beyond the obstruction becomes over-distended with air. Consequent loss of elasticity, and sometimes rupture of the alveoli, causes patches of emphysema and atelectasis. Unresolved atelectasis can lead to bronchiectasis either during or after the actual period of illness. Stasis of the thick pulmonary secretions predisposes to secondary infection which may progress to pneumonia. The resulting leukocytosis causes a mediastinal lymphadenopathy.

The severe coughing which occurs in an effort to expectorate the tenacious secretions causes vomiting and can rupture capillaries causing pulmonary haemorrhages and episodes of haemoptysis, facial oedema and petechiae of the face and neck and subconjunctival haemorrhages. Increased intracranial pressure with associated bradycardia and hypoxia occurs during the paroxysms of coughing which are often accompanied by periods of apnoea. This increased pressure can rupture cerebral vessels. Rarely, large intracranial haemorrhages with paralysis and death can result. Lengthy periods of apnoea can cause convulsions due to cerebral anoxia or asphyxia. Asphyxia and death may also be the result of airway obstruction by secretions and/or vomit. Brain damage can occur following prolonged deprivation of oxygen due to any of the above causes.

### 7.3 CLINICAL FEATURES

The clinical features of whooping cough can be divided into three main stages:

- The catarrhal stage occurs after the incubation period and lasts for about 2 weeks.
- The paroxysmal stage follows and can last for 5–6 weeks. In some cases it may persist for up to 12 weeks.
- The convalescent stage concludes the illness and extends for a further 2–4 weeks.

### The catarrhal stage

During this phase the features are those of any mild respiratory infection: coryza, cough, sneezing, watering eyes and a low grade pyrexia. These symptoms persist beyond the usual period for a mild infection and, as time progresses, the cough worsens, especially at night.

## The paroxysmal stage

As the cough becomes more severe it begins to occur in paroxysms. Each paroxysm consists of sudden episodic bursts of short rapid coughs which occur during expiration. During each paroxysm the child is momentarily deprived of oxygen and becomes red and then cyanosed. His eyes bulge and his tongue protrudes. If expiration is completely taken over by coughing, periods of apnoea may occur. At the end of each paroxysm a forceful inspiration occurs in an effort to replenish oxygen supplies. It is this forced intake of air which produces the characteristic high-pitched 'whooping' sound. This sound is less apparent and may not occur in infants under 6 months whose ability to cough is not fully developed. Several paroxysms can occur in quick succession until the child is able to expectorate the thick, tenacious sputum. The exertion of coughing may cause the child to vomit and leaves him sweating, tired and dazed. The paroxysms occur spontaneously but may also be precipitated by exertion or feeding.

## The convalescent stage

As the episodes of whooping and vomiting decrease the child can be said to be in the recovery phase. Paroxysms of less severe coughing may still occur but gradually the cough becomes more like that associated with a common cold. In some children exacerbations of the paroxysmal stage may occur for up to a year after the actual infection, usually associated with other respiratory illnesses.

## 7.4 MEDICAL MANAGEMENT

Only a small proportion of children with whooping cough are admitted to hospital. Even in the 1977–9 epidemic more than 97% of the affected children were cared for at home. Infants are among those most often hospitalized because the risk of aspyxia and other complications are more likely in this age group. Other children are admitted due to severe paroxysms or if serious complications have developed.

Whooping cough causes considerable stress to both child and parents. Parents are very anxious about the full recovery of their child. They often become exhausted from loss of sleep while caring for their child during the paroxysmal stage. Some children, especially those of one-parent families, may be admitted to relieve parental stress.

The most effective antimicrobial drug against various strains of *B. pertussis* is erythromycin. In 1986 studies showed that it:

- prevented whooping cough in susceptible contacts of the affected child;
- prevented the further onset of symptoms if given during the incubation period;
- reduced the severity of the illness if given during the catarrhal phase;
- prevented the secretion of *B. pertussis* from the affected child.

Oral salbutamol, 6 to 8 hourly, dilates the bronchioles and facilitates expectoration of the thick sputum during the paroxysmal stage. It reduces the incidence and duration of coughing and is usually given to children with severe paroxysms.

The incidence and duration of coughing in the paroxysmal stage may also be reduced by the use of corticosteroids. Oral betamethasone and intramuscular hydrocortisone succinate have both been effectively used. Because of the side-effects of corticosteroids they are usually only used for those children with life-threatening paroxysms.

## 7.5 NURSING CARE

### Assessment

*Breathing*

- Pattern of respiration. Does coughing interfere with expiration? Does the child become cyanosed or apnoeic at times?
- Cough. Does coughing occur in paroxysms? What is the frequency and duration of coughing? What does the cough sound like? Does any activity seem to precipitate coughing?
- Sputum. What is the colour and consistency of the sputum? Is expectoration difficult?

*Maintaining body temperature*

- Is the child pyrexial? Does he feel sweaty or dry?

## Eating and drinking

- Is the child able to eat and drink normally? Does this activity aggravate the cough?

## Elimination

- Is vomiting associated with cough? How often is this occurring?
- Is the child passing urine and faeces normally (i.e. is he dehydrated)?

## Rest and sleep

- Is this activity altered by coughing?
- Do the parents appear tired and lacking in sleep?

## Communication

- If the child has not been fully vaccinated, are the parents feeling guilty?

## Maintaining a safe environment

- Are any of the family, who may be visiting, at particular risk of contracting whooping cough themselves?

### Planning

The most crucial aspect of nursing care is to isolate the affected child in a cubicle and take protective precautions. Once a child has been exposed to *B. pertussis* neither active immunization nor passive immunization with hyperimmune globulin will provide protection. Isolation is the only way to prevent a hospital epidemic of whooping cough.

The cubicle should have humidified oxygen and suction available in case of periods of apnoea or asphyxia caused by inhalation of sputum or vomit. Suction should only be used periodically and with care as frequent and prolonged naso- and oropharyngeal suction often induces paroxysms of coughing.

The child should not be left alone because of the very real danger of airway obstruction. Resident or visiting parents

**Table 7.1** Care plan for an infant with whooping cough. Tim Simons aged 7 months has been admitted to the ward in the paroxysmal stage of whooping cough. He is the only child of young parents who feel unable to cope with his prolonged paroxyms of coughing. They report that 'he turns blue and stops breathing during his bouts of coughing'. On admission he is apyrexial but looks pale and tired. Although vomiting occurs at times after coughing he has not lost weight. His mother wishes to be resident

| Problem | Aim of care | Nursing intervention |
|---|---|---|
| Potential spread of infection | Those outside Tim's family will not contract his infection | Isolate in cubicle with infectious precautions<br>Limit visitors to close family<br>Advise family not to socialize with others on ward |
| Potential asphyxia and/or hypoxia due to airway obstruction by thick sputum or inhaled vomit | Tim will maintain:<br>a clear airway,<br>his colour;<br>his respiratory rate between 30 and 35/min;<br>his heart rate between 100 and 140/min | Stay with Tim at all times<br>Position on abdomen or side. Tip head of cot down<br>When Tim coughs:<br>tip him over your lap;<br>pat gently on back;<br>wipe sputum from nose and mouth<br>Record pulse and respiration hourly. Report any deviation<br>Give oxygen if Tim becomes cyanosed<br>Suction only if mucus is obstructing airway<br>Give clear feeds until Tim coughs without vomiting or cyanosis |

| Potential dehydration, malnutrition and weight loss due to vomiting after coughing episodes | Tim will receive at least 1200 ml daily and maintain his present weight (8 kg) | Offer Tim 100 ml of Dextrolyte at 2 hourly intervals half-an-hour after vomiting. Feed slowly. Sit upright during feeding<br>Record all intake and output<br>Weigh daily |
| Potential exhaustion due to severe coughing | Tim will rest for 2 h morning and afternoon and at least 8 h between 6 p.m. and 6 a.m. | Avoid waking or startling Tim<br>Plan rest periods morning and afternoon |
| Parental anxiety about Tim's progress | Tim's parents will understand his care and his condition | Encourage and teach parents how to handle Tim during paroxysms of coughing<br>Encourage and teach parents how to feed Tim<br>Explain that paroxysmal phase can last for 5–6 weeks |

should only be left alone with their child when the nurses is confident that they would know what to do in the event of such complications. Infants should always be positioned on their abdomens or side to minimize the danger of inhalation of sputum or vomit. The head of the cot should be tilted downwards.

Vital signs should be recorded at least 4 hourly. Respiratory rate, colour and heart rate are the most important observations. Episodes of apnoea and cyanosis are common during paroxysms of coughing but the exhaustion caused by frequent paroxysms may lead to respiratory failure. The nurse should also be alert for features of secondary respiratory infection and atelectasis. Frequent vomiting may lead to dehydration and malnutrition requiring parenteral nutrition. A careful account of fluid and calorie intake and fluid output should be maintained. Feeding should take place half-an-hour after vomiting wherever possible. Feeds should be small and given slowly to avoid exhaustion, coughing and further vomiting.

The child should be nursed at rest until apyrexial. In order to avoid exhaustion and precipitating paroxysms of coughing, nursing interventions should be carefully planned to allow for rest periods and to avoid waking the child. The nurse should also ensure that the child's parents have adequate physical and mental rest. She should try to relieve their anxieties by demonstrating how to handle the child during paroxysms. The length of the illness should be explained so that they recognize that the cough may persist for some time. Before the child is discharged they should also be told about the convalescent stage so that they do not have unrealistic expectations. They may feel guilty about the lack of failure of immunization and they should be allowed to express these feelings without feeling that they are being judged. Information about immunization of subsequent children may be appreciated.

Table 7.1 illustrates one care plan for a child with whooping cough.

7.6 HEALTH EDUCATION

The paediatric nurse has a role in providing parents with enough information about whooping cough immunization to enable them to make an informed decision about having their children vaccinated.

The Department of Health and Social Security recommends that the three-part course of combined pertussis–diphtheria–tetanus vaccine should be given between 4 and 12 months of age. There is some professional dispute about the safety and efficacy of the whooping cough vaccine. Several studies have reported a link between pertussis vaccine and brain damage in some infants. In 1981, the National Childhood Encephalopathy Study (NCES) reported that approximately 1 per 100 000 children receiving the full course of three injections of vaccine ran the risk of serious neurological reaction within 7 days of immunization. Infants most at risk are those who have a respiratory infection at the time of the immunization and those with a family history of fits. Careful questioning of the parents and examination of the infant always takes place before the first injection to exclude such infants from the immunization programme.

When the whooping cough vaccine was first introduced, it was insufficiently potent to provide protection. In 1968, the vaccine was reformulated and in 1977 its efficacy was reassessed. This new vaccine was found to provide adequate protection from *B. pertussis*, either by preventing the onset of whooping cough or by reducing the severity of the illness.

The opposite argument points out that whooping cough is a serious illness which itself can result in neurological damage due to cerebral anoxia or even death. In the 1977–9 epidemic, out of the 102 500 children who developed whooping cough, 5000 were admitted to hospital. Fifty of these required admission to intensive care units, 200 contracted secondary infections and 83 developed convulsions. Seventeen children, or approximately one in 6000, experienced lasting neurological damage and 27 children, or 1 in 4000, died. In 1982, 14 children died out of the 66 000 who contracted the infection, again showing a figure of approximately 1 in 4000.

The surge in the number of cases of whooping cough which occurred in 1978, and in 1982, coincided with the sharp drop in the rate of uptake of the vaccine. This appears to prove the efficacy of the vaccine. In order to protect those children who are too young for immunization and those in whom the vaccine is contraindicated there must be high herd immunity. This can only be achieved by an increased acceptance of the vaccine.

Current research is exploring the development of a new acellular anti-pertussis vaccine which aims to combine efficacy with greater safety.

# 8 Care of the toddler with croup

Croup is a nonspecific term given to a characteristic group of symptoms comprising hoarseness, 'barking cough', inspiratory stridor and varying degrees of respiratory distress.

Acute infections involving the larynx may also be described according to the primary area affected. Thus the term 'croup' may be given to acute laryngitis or laryngotracheobronchitis.

The characteristic features of croup appear as a result of laryngeal swelling and are of more concern in infants and small children than they are in older children. Babies and younger children have a greater chance of developing croup because of their susceptibility to infection of the respiratory tract. Also, their narrow airways may be severely compromised by any degree of inflammation.

Most children with croup have a mild infection which results in hoarseness and cough and lasts for about 7 days. However, complications and even death can occur. The more common complications such as otitis media, bronchiolitis and pneumonia are caused by spread of the infecting organism. Laryngeal obstruction is the most serious complication and causes the majority of deaths. Tracheostomy, which may be performed to relieve laryngeal obstruction, may lead to further complications. The severity of the disease is probably due to general factors affecting the child's susceptibility to infection rather than the power of the infecting organism.

8.1 AETIOLOGY

**Incidence and causative organisms**

The incidence of croup is related to the causative organism. The main aetiological agents are viruses and those most commonly isolated are influenza, A and B, parainfluenza 1, 2 and 3, and respiratory syncytial virus. Influenza and parainfluenza occur in epidemics during the winter and spring months (October and May). These epidemics tend to be more severe every 2 years and usually affect small children under 3 years. Respiratory syncytial virus tends only to affect the very young, particularly babies under 6 months. It is an endemic infection which can occur at any time of the year.

Rarely, croup can be caused by bacteria. In these cases it is associated with whooping cough or diptheria and caused by *Haemophilus influenza* or *Corynebacterium diptheriae*. Croup caused by these organisms is usually seen in older children, between the ages of 3 to 7 years.

**Transmission**

As a respiratory infection, croup is transmitted by inhalation of droplets. It is usually spread by the older child or adult who may have no noticeable signs of a viral infection. One episode of croup does not provide immunity although it does seem to modify the infection. The most severe symptoms usually occur with the initial infection and subsequent reinfection generally only results in a mild form of the condition.

Viral agents are intracellular and, once inhaled, spread to adjacent areas. The entire respiratory tract is potentially at risk. Clinically, the specific area involved, in this case the larynx, is due to the relatively narrow larynx of small children.

8.2 PATHOPHYSIOLOGY

The infecting organism causes an inflammatory reaction in the upper respiratory tract. As a result, the mucous glands in this area swell and secrete more mucus. The inflammation and increased secretions prevent ciliary function in the affected area. Loss of ciliary activity presents the humdification of inspired air. The body's natural mechanisms for humidifying air is further aggravated by the increased secretions blocking the nose and nasopharynx and forcing the child to breathe through his mouth. In order to saturate the incoming air, water has to be evaporated from the lower respiratory tract. The child is already losing an increased amount of water due to pyrexia. He also has a decreased fluid intake as the nasal obstruction impairs feeding, especially in the infant who relies on sucking to take in food and fluid. All these physiological changes result in a decreased amount of body fluid which causes the production of thickened secretions. The presence of these thick secretions in the lower respiratory tract is irritating and the child begins to cough to expel the mucus and clear the tracheobronchial tree.

Young children have difficulty expelling the increased secretions in the nasal area and the infection descends the respiratory tract to cause oedema of the pharynx, larynx, trachea and bronchi. Even a small degree of swelling in these areas narrows the lumen of a small child's airway sufficiently to cause dyspnoea. Laryngeal oedema at the level of the cricoid cartilage, which is the narrowest part of the small child's larynx, causes inspiratory stridor (a harsh, shrill sound heard with every intake of air). Oedema of the vocal cords causes hoarseness.

The child now has a swollen, narrowed upper respiratory tract and increased viscous secretions in the lower part of his respiratory system. Consequently, respiratory effort is increased which, together with the raised metabolic rate due to pyrexia, causes an increase in oxygen consumption and cardiac workload. This may cause exhaustion in the smaller child and as respiratory effort decreases with tiredness, the obstruction of the airway is exacerbated and may ultimately result in respiratory arrest.

8.3 CLINICAL FEATURES

The onset of croup is usually gradual and follows what appears to be a simple upper respiratory tract infection with a runny nose, mild pyrexia and slight loss of appetite. After 3 or 4 days these features progress and the first stages of laryngeal involvement become apparent – cough, dyspnoea, stridor and hoarseness. At the same time the pyrexia increases. These features usually last for 3 to 5 days. At the end of this time the child either beings to improve spontaneously or his symptoms worsen as the infection increases.

Respiratory distress becomes more evident with intercostal and substernal retractions, nasal flaring and use of the accessory muscles of respiration. Expiration may be particularly laboured and difficult. This increased respiratory effort is accompanied by an increased pulse rate and also causes the child to have difficulty in feeding. The increased secretions present in the lower respiratory tract may be audible, causing coarse rattling sounds.

If the inflammation of the upper respiratory tract continues, airway obstruction begins to develop. The child becomes anxious, irritable and restless, and pallor cyanosis results from the retention of carbon dioxide and hypoxia. The inspiratory stridor becomes more obvious and the child becomes cold and clammy as he struggles to take in air.

## 8.4 INVESTIGATIONS

The diagnosis of croup is usually made by the history of a few days' mild illness followed by the appearance of the characteristic features of laryngeal swelling.

Blood tests will show little evidence of infection. The white cell count may be normal or only slightly raised and an increased $pO_2$ may not be evident in the early stages of the condition. A decreased $pCO_2$ is only seen as a late sign when respiration is severely impaired by obstruction.

An X-ray of the neck will show swelling of the laryngeal part of the pharynx at the area of the cricoid cartilage, with normal structures above this level.

## 8.5 MEDICAL MANAGEMENT

The treatment of croup aims to maintain a clear airway and ensure adequate gaseous exchange. Children who have only mild clinical features can usually be managed at home with symptomatic treatment such as rest and humidified air until the cough has subsided. Hospitalization is indicated for those children who are particularly susceptible to laryngeal obstruction. The children at risk are those with more severe features of croup and those who naturally have narrow airways. They can be identified as children with:

- progressive stridor and dyspnoea;
- a hyperpyrexia and a toxic appearance;
- restlessness, anxiety and pallor or cyanosis;
- small diameter airways such as infants under 1 year, in whom 1 mm of oedema can halve the lumen of the larynx;
- congential subglottic stenosis;
- a history of previous airway instrumentation and/or ventilation which may have damaged the airways and caused scarring and fibrosis.

For the children, hospitalization provides constant observation to ensure a clear airway and the facilities and equipment for tracheostomy and/or ventilation if necessary. Adequate gaseous exchange can be aided by humidification and the provision of an environment which is rich in oxygen. Arterial blood gases and pH can be monitored to assess the efficacy of this together with repeated chest and lateral neck X-rays.

Reduction and loosening of the thick secretions can be helped further by adequate hydration. As the child cannot take sufficient oral fluids, and aspiration is a risk if he is forced to do so, intravenous fluids are commenced. Approximately 250–300 ml/kg/24 h is given to allow for the increased metabolic rate. Care must be taken to ensure that the child's circulation is not further stressed by fluid overload. A cardiac monitor may be used to enable constant observation of cardiac rate and rhythm.

Severe obstruction may necessitate tracheostomy and/or ventilation. The decision to insert an artificial airway is based upon several factors. These criteria include:

- Increasing agitation and anxiety of the child.
- $pO_2$ of 50 mmHg even with supplemental oxygen.
- $pCO_2$ of 55 mmHg.
- Increasing cardiac and respiratory rates indicating exhaustion. (In small infants this may be demonstrated by apnoeic attacks.)
- Progressive and worsening signs of laryngeal obstruction.

The artificial airway may be formed by a tracheostomy or intubation. Intubation with the use of a nasotracheal tube is the method of choice. Once the laryngeal swelling has subsided the child can be extubated. Spontaneous breathing should follow. If the child's airway remains obstructed once the acute inflammation has settled, usually due to stenosis of the airways due to other problems, a tracheostomy may be necessary. Supplemental oxygen and humidification should continue with the use of a tracheostomy mask or by direct attachment to a mechanical ventilator. Improvement is often immediate although mild sedation may be necessary to enable him to adjust to the tracheostomy or nasotracheal tube. Removal of the tube can be performed as soon as the child's vital signs return to normal and his secretions have lessened.

Medications are mostly ineffective or contraindicated in children with viral croup. Antipyretics may be given for any pyrexia over 38°C to prevent further dryness of secretions and increased respiratory and cardiac effort. Intravenous ampicillin (150 mg/kg/24 h) may be prescribed for those children with suspected bacterial croup.

## 8.6 NURSING CARE

### Assessment

#### Breathing

- What is the child's respiratory rate and rhythm?
- Is there any nasal flaring or abnormal chest movements?
- Does the child seem pale or cyanosed?
- Are there any abnormal breath sounds? How may these sounds be described? During which part of respiration do they occur?
- Is the child coughing? What kind of cough is it?
- Is the child able to expel any secretions? What do the secretions look like?
- Has the child had any breathing problems before? How were these treated?

#### Maintaining body temperature

- What is the child's temperature?
- Does his skin feel hot and dry or cold and clammy?

#### Eating and drinking

- How has this illness affected the child's usual feeding pattern?

*Rest and sleep*

- Has the respiratory distress disturbed the child's normal rest and sleep pattern?
- Does he appear restless or exhausted?

*Communication*

- Has the child become more irritable or anxious with the course of the disease?

**Planning**

The most important aspect of nursing care for the child with croup is close observation to allow for the early recognition of laryngeal obstruction. Emergency equipment for performing a tracheostomy or intubation should be in readiness until respiratory distress has ceased. Relief of dyspnoea can be provided by nursing the child in a cool, high humidity environment with oxygen. He should be allowed to rest as much as possible. A small child, frighted by his illness and hospitalization, needs the security of his parents' presence or a nurse to enable him to achieve physical and mental rest. Parents will also need reassurance as they will be frightened by their child's illness, especially if an artificial airway is necessary, and they may feel guilty that they did not recognize the severity of their child's condition.

Although the child who requires a tracheostomy or intubation may experience immediate relief of symptoms, he may become more frightened when he realizes that he cannot speak or cry. At this time he continues to need emotional support by the constant presence of parents or nursing staff. Close observation should also continue as airway obstruction can still occur due to mucous plugs. For this reason suction should be carried out at frequent intervals following the injection of 0.5–2 ml of sterile normal saline into the tube to loosen the secretions. Infants can occlude their tracheostomy or endotracheal tube with their chins so a small roll should be placed under his shoulders to extend his neck.

The child with a tracheostomy is at risk from accidental removal of the tube and irritation of the wound site causing secondary infection. Tracheal dilators and a spare tracheostomy

**Table 8.1** Care of the toddler with croup. Helen Cox, aged 18 months, is admitted to the ward with croup. She is accompanied by her parents. On admission she looks flushed and anxious. Her temperature is 39°C, her respirations 40/min and her pulse rate 140/min. She is obviously dyspnoeic and chest retractions are marked. She has an inspiratory stridor and a hoarse cry. Her parents report that she developed a cold 4 days previously and that her condition has gradually deteriorated over the last 24 h. During this deterioration she has been unable to eat and has taken very little fluid. Helen is placed in an oxygen tent and an intravenous infusion of dextrase/saline at 30 ml/h is commenced. She becomes very upset during these procedures and is obviously frightened. Mrs Cox would like to be resident

| Problem | Aim of care | Nursing intervention |
|---|---|---|
| Potential obstruction of airway due to excessive thick secretions | (a) To loosen and liquefy secretions <br> (b) To observe for signs of obstruction <br> (c) To prepare for the insertion of an artificial airway | Nurse in an oxygen tent with high humidification <br> Inform doctor if Helen develops: <br> restlessness <br> increased stridor or chest retractions <br> nasal flaring <br> pallor or cyanosis <br> Wipe inside of tent frequently to clear condensation and facilitate observation <br> Check that the emergency trolley is nearby and in working order |
| Respiratory distress (respiratory rate = 40/min, heart rate = 140/min) | To reduce Helen's respiratory effort and restore her respiratory rate to 25–30/min and her heart rate to 100–120/min | Nurse in 40% oxygen <br> Monitor pulse and respirations hourly until stable <br> Inform doctor if respiratory rate exceeds 40/min or pulse rate above 160/min <br> Plan care to allow Helen uninterrupted rest periods |

**Table 8.1** contd

| Problem | Aim of care | Nursing intervention |
|---|---|---|
| Increased metabolic rate due to pyrexia | To reduce Helen's oxygen consumption by reducing her temperature to 37–38°C | Administer Calpol 5 ml 4 hourly as prescribed when Helen's temperature is over 38°C<br>Nurse exposed<br>Monitor temperature hourly |
| Potential dehydration as unable to take adequate food and fluids | To ensure Helen's skin and mucous membranes remain moist and healthy and that she receives an intake of at least 1500 ml/24 h | Monitor infusion running at prescribed rate<br>Monitor all intake and output<br>Observe for signs of dehydration:<br>  dry, inelastic skin<br>  oliguria<br>  constipation<br>  weight loss<br>Give mouth care 2–4 hourly while taking nothing by mouth |
| Helen is crying due to the unfamiliar environment | To keep Helen calm | Encourage mother to stay beside Helen and participate in her care<br>Give Helen her usual comforter/toy<br>Spend time with Helen and her mother to establish a rapport with Helen<br>Be available to stay with Helen when mother is not available |
| Mr and Mrs Cox are anxious about Helen's condition | For Mr and Mrs Cox to be able to talk about their worries | Explain the reasons for Helen's condition and treatment<br>Give them time to express their concerns |

tube should be kept at the cotside. The area around the tube should be kept clean and dry with a sterile dressing, and the tracheostomy tapes changed daily and tied securely. Table 8.1 illustrates one care plan for a toddler with croup.

When the child is ready for discharge the parents should be taught how to cope with any future attacks of croup. They should also be advised to keep their child indoors for 1 week after discharge and to try to keep him away from those who have a known infection. He can feed normally but should have extra clear fluids for the first week. They should be warned that coughing or hoarseness may linger for a week or two.

8.7 HEALTH EDUCATION

As croup is a relatively common respiratory infection in the under 3s and most of these children have a mild form of the condition which can be managed at home, parents should be advised on ways to relieve their child's breathlessness and stridor. They can be advised that if their child develops hoarseness and a croupy cough following a cold they should:

- Sit with their child in a steamy bathroom. This can be achieved by running hot water in the bath or shower and allowing the closed room to fill with steam. This usually gives quick relief to the noisy breathing, but if the child has not improved in 10 min, the doctor should be contacted.
- If the breathing improves, continued relief can be given by ensuring that the child's bedroom is warm but well ventilated.
- If he appears feverish give him any paediatric mixture that is recommended to relieve fever (e.g. Calpol). Let him wear only a nappy providing he is not shivering.
- Give the child a bottle or cup of his favourite drink every hour when he is awake.
- Position the child upright in his cot or bed. The older child can be propped upright on pillows but a baby will be safer in an infant seat.
- If the child continues to have noisy breathing keep a close watch on him. The doctor should be contacted if his
  breathlessness or fever increases;
  behaviour becomes very restless and agitated;
  lips or fingertips become bluish;
  chest below the ribs appears to sink in with each breath.

# 9  Care of the pre-school child with asthma

Asthma is a common disorder which is difficult to define precisely. It is caused by a variety of factors and the breathlessness which results from it may vary from a brief attack of mild wheezing to prolonged life-threatening episodes of acute dyspnoea as seen in status asthmaticus. The most commonly used definition of asthma describes it as a chronic recurrent condition which is characterized by wide variations to airflow in intrapulmonary airways over short periods of time. It is basically an allergic reaction which is characterized by spasm of the smooth muscle lining the bronchi and bronchioles, hypersecretion of mucus and mucosal oedema. These changes cause narrowing of the airways. 'Asthma' is a Greek word meaning 'whistling' and is descriptive of this condition because the large volumes of air which pass through the narrowed airways produce a whistling or wheezing sound.

Children with asthma fall into three main groups: 75% have infrequent attacks which are usually confined to episodes of viral upper respiratory tract infections; approximately 22% have more frequent and severe attacks which are precipitated by a variety of factors. These two groups of children usually have normal lung function between attacks. The remaining group of children are usually short, thin children who have chest deformities and permanent abnormal lung function due to their severe bronchoconstriction.

Whatever the frequency or severity of a child's asthma, his family experience anxiety and stress in relation to the fear caused by the child's symptoms during an attack, the prognosis of the condition and the possible inherited cause of the disorder.

9.1 AETIOLOGY

**Incidence**

Between 10 and 30% of the population have had wheezing at some time in their lives. In most of these cases, wheezing will be as a result of a temporary abnormal narrowing of the airways as a transient response to a nonspecific viral infection. An asthmatic is someone who shows sustained or recurrent features and studies suggest that about 5% of children in the UK are affected. The USA shows a similar prevalence but in smaller communities such as Lapland and North American Indian settlements the incidence is much lower. In Australia and New Zealand the prevalence is higher at 6–7%.

About 15–20% of asthmatic children develop symptoms during their first year of life but the majority of children develop the characteristic features of the condition between the ages of 2 and 5 years. It is twice as common in boys than girls and boys tend to show more severe symptoms. More than half the children with asthma will grow out of it completely and thus these sex differences disappear at puberty.

Approximately 75% of children with asthma will have a family history of some form of allergy. An immediate family member or the child himself usually shows other manifestations of allergy such as eczema, hay fever or urticaria. The importance of genetic factors in the incidence of asthma can be shown by the high incidence of asthma among the inhabitants of the island of Tristan da Cunha which can be traced back to the original settlers among whom were three asthmatic women. However, genetic disposition is not the only factor involved in the development of asthma, environmental factors are also involved. Racial groups who have a low prevalence of asthma and live in isolated rural environments increase their likelihood of developing asthma when they move to an urban environment, probably because they increase their exposure to allergens such as house dust mites or fungal spores, or to infectious organisms.

Asthma attacks can occur at any time of the year. Seasonal asthma during June and July is usually related to allergy to grass pollen and often is associated with rhinitus and conjunctivitis. Asthmatics may be worse in winter due to viral infections which tend to be more prominent at this time.

**Causative factors**

Asthma can be caused by intrinsic or extrinsic factors. Extrinsic asthma is caused by an identifiable external stimulus and is the type of asthma mostly affecting children. Intrinsic asthma, or that which has no specific stimulus, is usually seen when asthma begins during adulthood. Extrinsic asthma may be triggered off in six main ways:

- allergens
- emotion
- environmental changes
- exercise
- infections
- irritants

*Allergens*

Allergies may be acquired to airborne particles, dietary items and to drugs. The most common and potent allergen is domestic dust which harbours the house-dust mite, *Dermatophagoides pteronyssinus*. These microscopic insects thrive on skin scales and are, therefore, found in particular abundance in bedrooms, in feather pillows, mattresses and down-filled quilts.

Household pets may also be a cause of allergy. Cats are most often the cause as allergens may be present in their saliva, urine and fur.

Food allergy tends to cause eczema and gastrointestinal upsets rather than asthma but those children who develop asthma due to a food intolerance are often those with severe asthma. The foodstuffs most likely to cause allergy are milk, eggs, nuts and wheat. Food additives, such as tartrazine (the yellow dye widely used in the colouring of drinks, sweets and medications), are also common causes of allergy.

*Emotion*

Emotional factors alone do not cause asthma. However, in individuals with asthma, emotion may affect the way in which the bronchi and bronchioles respond to various stimuli and to medication. Emotions which alter bronchial response include anger, fear, stress and hilarity. It is thought that overbreathing, which occurs in all these types of emotion, may be the trigger factor. In an asthmatic child, fear and anxiety may stem from the emotional response of his parents towards him and his condition.

## Environmental changes

Changes in the weather can affect some asthmatic children. Climate affects plant growth, and pollen and seed dispersion may alter the child's frequency of attacks. Cold air can increase wheezing but cold, pure mountain air may decrease it. Changes in humidity can also affect wheezing. Dry heat from electric fires, for example, is an irritant to asthmatics.

## Exercise

Children whose asthmatic attacks are induced by any of the causative factors will usually be made worse by participating in vigorous exercise. Vigorous exercise produces bronchoconstriction and wheezing in most asthmatics but usually does not progress into an actual asthmatic attack unless another precipitating factor is involved. The type of exercise influences the degree of narrowing in the airways, running usually causes severe wheezing whereas swimming is least likely to cause problems. It seems that this difference depends on the fact that cooling of the airways during hyperventilation is the main cause of bronchoconstriction. In indoor swimming pools any hyperventilation caused by vigorous exercise is in a warm humid atmosphere which prevents an asthmatic response.

## Infection

Most asthmatic children wheeze more during the winter months usually due to viral respiratory tract infections, especially influenza. Infection in the bronchi and bronchioles always causes mucosal oedema and hypersecretion of mucus but in susceptible children it also causes, or exacerbates, bronchospasm and asthma.

## Irritants

Children with asthma show an increased reaction to inhaled

irritants and develop bronchoconstriction when subject to low concentrations of irritant agents. Tobacco smoke and dust are common irritants within the home environment but asthmatic children choosing a career should be aware that certain occupations would expose them to other irritant inhalants. Agents such as proteolytic enzymes, laboratory animals and insects, and grain or flour dust are particularly likely to cause problems.

Asthma can also be drug-induced: β-blocking agents such as atenolol and propanalol, often cause bronchoconstriction in asthmatic children even when given locally. Salicylates and non-steroidal anti-inflammatory agents can cause airway obstruction but this reaction is usually confined to adults. Occasionally, drugs used to treat asthma, such as aminophylline and sodium cromoglycate, can, paradoxically, cause bronchoconstriction. Nebulized hypotonic solutions, which result if medications are mixed with water instead of saline, can also induce bronchospasm.

### 9.2 PATHOPHYSIOLOGY

The asthmatic child has hyper-reactive airways. The respiratory system normally has a complicated system of responses including the cough reflex to protect it against any potentially damaging substances which may be inhaled. These reflexes, which are mainly transmitted by the vagus nerve, are more sensitive in asthmatics and the resulting responses are exaggerated. As yet there is no known reason why this hyperactivity occurs. It could be caused by abnormal epithelial cells in the lining of the airways either transmitting an increased impulse or over-responding to an impulse. Alternatively, the fault may be with the receptors which receive the impulse or with the motor system which relays the impulse.

Many of the factors which induce this hyper-reactive response do so by being directly toxic or irritant, or by eliciting the immune response. The immune response is brought about by the action of a specific type of antibody or immunoglobulin which is named immunoglobulin E (IgE).

IgE is produced by the body in response to a specific substance and becomes firmly attached to the outer surface of the mast cells which line the inner layer of the respiratory system. The mast cells contain granules which consist of toxic chemicals, amines, which when released cause the characteristic

Normal bronchus

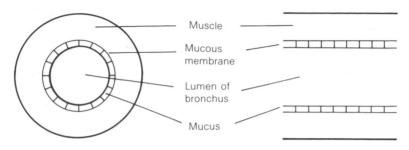

Asthmatic bronchus

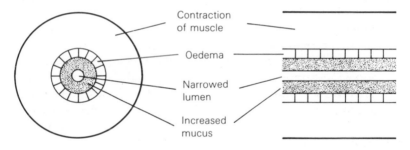

**Figure 9.1** Bronchial changes in asthma.

bronchoconstriction, oedema and hypersecretion of mucus. When the individual next comes into contact with the substance to which he is allergic – the allergen – the IgE reacts to it and the mast cells releases amines into the surrounding tissues.

Whatever the cause of asthma attacks, the mechanisms responsible for the obstructive features are:

- Oedema of the mucous membranes.
- Accumulation of increased secretions from the mucous glands.
- Spasm of the smooth muscle of the bronchi and bronchioles.

Inflammation of the mucous membrane lining of the respiratory system causes swelling and hypersecretion of the mucous glands. Accumulated secretions stimulate the cough reflex.

The smooth muscle of the respiratory tract is arranged in spiral bundles around the airway. Spasm of the muscle causes narrowing and shortening of the airways and resistance to airflow. During normal respiration the bronchi dilate and lengthen during inspiration and constrict and shorten during expiration. Thus the changes which occur during asthma attacks produce difficulty in breathing, particularly during expiration (Figure 9.1). Expired air is forced through the narrowed airways and the remainder is trapped in the lungs. As the bronchospasm continues the volume of trapped air increases forcing the individual to hyperventilate in an effort to take in sufficient air and maintain gaseous exchange. Hyperventilation increases the elastic recoil of the lungs and decreases the efficiency of the respiratory muscles. The alveoli overinflate with trapped air and cause bronchiolar dilation. This helps gaseous exchange but requires even more energy during inspiration to allow air to enter the lung tissues which are already distended. The fight for air causes fatigue and sweating. As breathing becomes less effective, oxygen consumption and cardiac output increase and the child becomes increasingly dyspnoeic, cyanotic and tachypnoeic. Coughing also becomes less effective and there is a very real danger of asphyxia caused by a plug of mucus. Eventually carbon dioxide retention, hypoxia and respiratory acidosis occurs causing respiratory failure and death.

## 9.3 CLINICAL FEATURES

Children with asthma will have varying features according to the severity and frequency of their asthma attacks. There are three main clinical patterns:

- acute asthma;
- chronic asthma;
- severe acute asthma.

### Acute asthma

The onset and length of acute asthmatic attacks varies according to their cause. Episodes caused by upper respiratory tract infections usually begin insiduously and tend to be prolonged.

Attacks which are induced by a specific allergen are generally acute and brief once the allergen has been removed. Whatever the cause, an acute episode of asthma begins with a dry non-productive, paroxysmal cough as a reflex reaction to the increased secretions produced by the bronchial oedema. As the secretions become more excessive, the cough produces plugs of clear, tenacious sputum. The older child becomes obviously dyspnoeic and appears to struggle to breathe. He sits upright with hunched shoulders and arms braced on the bed or chair and can be seen to be using his shoulder and neck muscles to facilitate respiration. Expiration, which is accompanied by wheezing, is particularly difficult. The child is pale with peripheral cyanosis and is sweaty and frightened. The abdominal breathing and rapid respiratory rate of normal infants and small children makes dyspnoea more difficult to visualize in younger children. These children show intercostal and suprasternal retractions and are restless, fidgety and irritable with a wheezy cry. Children who have acute asthmatic attacks usually have normal respiratory function between attacks.

**Chronic asthma**

Children with chronic asthma who are subject to repeated asthmatic attacks have physical deformities due to the repeated, prolonged attacks of hyperventilation. The thoracic cavity becomes fixed in the position that occurs in the fight for breath during an attack. The diaphragm becomes depressed and the shoulders elevate making the chest look barrel-shaped. Because of this fixed chest position the child has permanently to use his neck, shoulder and abdominal muscles to aid respiration. His respiratory function is always abnormal with a poor expiratory volume and a consistency raised $pCO_2$.

**Severe acute asthma**

Occasionally, for no specific reason, children with asthma develop an attack which does not respond to the usual treatment. At one time this situation was termed 'status asthmaticus'. Severe attacks are prolonged and increase in severity with time. The child is acutely dyspnoeic, and can only speak or cry in gasps, if at all. The profuse sweating which develops during the struggle for breath may cause dehydration. He has a shallow, irregular tachypnoea which, together with a tachycardia, cyanosis and diminishing consciousness, indicate deterioration and potential asphyxia.

## 9.4 INVESTIGATIONS

Children which chronic asthma usually develop features during infancy. A history of two to three attacks of severe wheezing and a family history of allergies is usually diagnostic of asthma providing other rarer causes of wheezing such as an inhaled foreign body or congenital obstruction to the lower trachea or bronchi have been eliminated.

A diagnosis of asthma can be confirmed in children of 4 years and over who have a history of recurrent episodes of coughing, wheezing and breathlessness with the use of a peak flow meter. In these children a low reading which improves by more than 20% after bronchodilators allows a positive diagnosis. A family history of allergy strengthens any doubtful result. An exercise provocation test can be given to children over 3 years to discover if running causes a fall in peak flow and/or brings on wheezing. In some respiratory function laboratories this exercise test has now been replaced by measuring the child's response to hyperventilation in a cold atmosphere.

A skin prick test can be used to identify allergies. A minute amount of common allergens (house dust mite, pollens, animal fur) is injected into the superficial layers of the epidermis. A weal develops at the injection site if a specific IgE antibody is present. This test does not diagnose asthma as it can only identify those children who have a tendency to develop allergies, but it can help to confirm a diagnosis in the child who demonstrates other asthmatic features.

## 9.5 MEDICAL MANAGEMENT

The management of asthma is two-fold. The child with asthma needs day to day long-term management to eliminate or avoid the causative factor(s), and the child with an acute attack needs early recognition and treatment of this medical emergency.

## Long-term control

### Allergen control

Avoidance of obvious precipitating factors such as animals is advised for those children with specific allergens. However, there are often other unknown factors that cannot be dealt with so easily. Most children with allergies are sensitive to pollen or house dust mites which are almost impossible to avoid. There is little evidence to show that desensitization is useful in allergic asthma.

### Medications

Disodium cromoglyate inhibits the release of chemical mediators from the mast cells. It is thus a prophylatic drug and should be taken regularly. It may take up to 4 weeks to take effect.

β stimulants are useful for the majority of asthmatic children who do not require medication continuously. Salbutamol or terbutaline, for example, can be inhaled at the onset of symptoms or if symptom-provoking situations occur. These bronchodilator drugs act quickly and their effect can last for up to 6 h.

Inhaled steroids such as budesonide or beclomethasone can also be used for prophylaxis. They have the added advantage of potentiating the action of any bronchodilators and can be usefully used concurrently with β stimulants. Some children with chronic asthma which is resistant to treatment require oral prednisolone. In such cases, it is given on alternate days to decrease the serious side-effects, such as retardation of growth, that can occur in children.

### Physiotherapy

For children with chronic asthma, breathing exercises are useful to prevent hyperinflation and to improve the strength of respiratory muscles. Sit ups and leg exercises aid expiration by strengthening abdominal muscles. Although vigorous exercise is not usually possible, moderate exercise such as cricket, rounders, short sprints and swimming is advantageous as it promotes fitness and peer interaction. Children with exercise-induced asthma can prevent an attack with a prior inhalation of a $\beta$ stimulant.

*Control of other factors*

Children who develop asthma due to emotional factors must have adequate explanation and control of their condition if they are to feel confident. Parents must also feel in control of their child's illness so that their anxiety is not transmitted to the child. They should not over-protect the child or allow him to use his illness to manipulate them.

Children prone to respiratory infections should be helped to lose weight if necessary, avoid excessive tiredness and, where possible, avoid others with infections.

**Management of acute asthma**

Deaths from asthma occur when the severity of the situation has not been fully appreciated. Hospitalization is recommended if cyanosis is present of if the child does not quickly respond to his usual home medication and nebulized salbutamol.

On admission a high percentage of humidified oxygen should be given to achieve a $pO_2$ of about 150 mmHg and reverse anaerobic metabolism. Parenteral fluids are usually required to replace insensible fluid lost due to tachypnoea. Aminophylline (5–8 mg/kg body wt.) can be added to the infusion every 6 h together with nebulized salbutamol 2 hourly. If the child has been treated with steroids in the last 6 months, intravenous hydrocortisone 4 mg/kg 2 hourly may be required. Children who do not respond to this treatment and continue to deteriorate will also need assisted ventilation. When $pO_2$ and $pCO_2$ return to normal levels ventilation can be gradually discontinued. When the child has been weaned off the ventilator and his peak flow rate is at lest 75% of the normal range for his age, height and weight, his drugs can be gradually reduced until he is taking the treatment he will have at home.

9.6 NURSING CARE

**Assessment**

*Breathing*

- What is the child's rate and pattern of breathing?
- Is he cyanotic?
- Is he using any of the accessory muscles of respiration?
- What position does he adopt to help him breathe?
- Is the child's cough dry or productive?
- If sputum is expectorated, what is its colour and consistency?

*Maintaining body temperature*

- Is the child pyrexial?

*Eating and drinking*

- Has the child had difficulty eating and drinking due to his breathlessness?
- Does he have an allergy to any foodstuffs?

*Elimination*

- Is the child perspiring?
- Do his skin and mucous membranes appear dry?

*Rest and sleep*

- Has breathlessness prevented this activity?
- Does the child appear restless and agitated?

*Communication*

- Can the child speak while he is breathless? (Is the infant able to cry normally?)

*Maintaining a safe environment*

- Does the child have any known precipitating factors that might be present in hospital?
- Does the child or parents know what caused this attack?

**Planning**

Before the child is admitted, his bed or cot area should be prepared with oxygen and suction equipment. The resuscitation trolley should be nearby. Any potential allergens, feather pillows, flowers or furry, stuffed toys, should be removed.

One of the most important aspects of caring for a child with severe asthma is to allay the child's anxiety. The child with severe asthma is in acute distress, exhausted and frightened due to his dyspnoea. The constant presence of his parents and a calm and competent nurse will help to reassure him. The parents also need reassurance. They will be upset and anxious about their child's condition and may feel guilty in case they are in some way responsible for the disorder. Parental anxiety is often transmitted to the child who becomes even more fearful. The presence of a senior nurse who can explain what is happening and respond quickly and calmly to the child's needs will thus help the child and his parents.

The child should be positioned upright to help his dyspnoea and given a high percentage of humidified oxygen. The younger child can be given humidified oxygen via a mist tent provided that this does not distress him. The extreme respiratory effort required during an asthmatic attack, and the consequent inability to rest and sleep, can cause acute exhaustion. For this reason, nursing the child on his mother's lap may be preferable to the oxygen tent if the child feels more secure.

The child should be continually observed for signs of deterioration which could indicate respiratory failure and for any toxic effects of treatment. Aminophylline can cause hypotension, tachycardia, tremor and apprehension due to its action on the sympathetic nervous system. A record of intake and output should be kept to ensure adequate hydration and to liquefy secretions. Insensible loss should be taken into account as sweating may be considerable. Oral fluid can be encouraged when the child is less breathless. Table 9.1 lists the care plan for a typical case history of severe asthma.

Once the acute phase is over the cause of the attack should be ascertained so that the parents may be given appropriate advice about the prevention of further attacks.

**Table 9.1** Care plan for the pre-school child with severe asthma. Hitesh Mahmoud, aged 4 years, is admitted to the ward with an acute attack of asthma. He is accompanied by his father as his mother has had to stay at home with his baby brother, aged 3 weeks. On admission, Hitesh is acutely breathless, pale, sweating, restless and anxious. He is wheezing and has a rattling cough, although unable to expectorate. He is apyrexial with a pulse rate of 130/min and a respiratory rate of 35/min. His father reports that Hitesh has had previous asthmatic attacks when he has had an infection or been in contact with cats or dogs but he does not know the reason for this episode. He admits that Hitesh feels neglected since the new baby arrived. Hitesh has never required hospitalization before

| Problem | Aim of care | Nursing intervention |
|---|---|---|
| Severe respiratory distress (respiratory rate = 35/min) due to bronchospasm | To reduce Hitesh's respiratory distress and reduce respiratory rate to at least 24/min | Administer aminophylline infusion as prescribed<br>Nurse in an upright position in an oxygen tent if tolerated<br>Observe respiratory rate and degree of distress half-hourly<br>Report increased agitation, respirations, confusion or cyanosis |
| Hitesh and his father are anxious due to Hitesh's condition and the unfamiliar surroundings | To help them understand what is happening and become less anxious | Stay with Hitesh<br>Explain all care and how it will help Hitesh get better<br>Provide all care calmly<br>Encourage Dad to stay and help with Hitesh's care |
| Potential asphyxia due to bronchial obstruction by mucous plugs | To liquefy secretions and enable Hitesh to expectorate | Give humidified oxygen<br>Ensure IVI running to prescribed rate (50 ml/h)<br>Encourage oral fluids when Hitesh is less breathless<br>Chest physiotherapy |

**Table 9.1** contd

| Problem | Aim of care | Nursing intervention |
|---|---|---|
| Potential signs of shock due to sympathetic stimulation by bronchodilators | To observe Hitesh for tremor, hypotension or tachycardia | Record half-hourly pulse and blood pressure<br>Report any abnormalities<br>Observe Hitesh for tremor |
| Exhaustion due to prolonged respiratory distress causing inability to rest | To allow Hitesh to rest between periods of essential care | Plan care to allow 20 min rest between observations<br>Maintain quiet, restful atmosphere<br>Allow Hitesh to sit on Dad's lap if unable to rest in oxygen tent |
| Potential dehydration due to sweating and increased metabolic rate | To ensure Hitesh has an intake of at least 1.5 litres | Monitor IVI as above<br>Encourage oral fluids when able<br>Record all intake and output (allow 300 ml insensible loss) |
| Potential maternal separation anxiety | To provide Hitesh with constant reminders of his mother | Encourage Mum to telephone Hitesh daily<br>Ask parents to bring something of mother's for Hitesh to keep<br>Keep to Hitesh's normal home routine as far as possible |

Forty-eight hours later Hitesh is much improved. He is only slightly wheezy and can play in the ward without becoming short of breath. His infusion has been discontinued and he is now having nebulized salbutamol 4 hourly as required and disodium cromoglyate via a spinhaler three times a day. Preparations can be made for him to return home

| Problem | Aim of care | Nursing intervention |
|---|---|---|
| Wheeziness | For wheeziness to be reduced to a minimum | Administer salbutamol as prescribed 4 hourly when wheezy |
| Parents may lack knowledge of Hitesh's medication | For Mr and Mrs Mahmoud to be able to administer Hitesh's drugs with confidence and safety | Explain need for salbutamol inhaler when Hitesh is wheezy<br>Warn that salbutamol should not be given more than 4 hourly<br>Explain that Intal is a preventative drug and must be given regularly<br>Demonstrate the administration of inhalers and allow the parents to participate |
| Mr and Mrs Mahmoud may not fully understand the precipitating factors of Hitesh's asthma | For Mr and Mrs Mahmoud to recognize precipitating factors and know how to prevent further attacks | Discuss prevention of infection:<br>avoid contact with those with respiratory infection<br>ensure adequate rest<br>seek medical advice as soon as infection occurs<br>well-balanced diet |

**Table 9.1** contd

| Problem | Aim of care | Nursing intervention |
|---------|-------------|----------------------|
| | | Discuss psychological factors: involve Hitesh in caring for the baby do not allow baby to alter Hitesh's routine give Hitesh plenty of reassurance that he is still loved do not allow Hitesh to use his asthma as a means of achieving attention |
| Potential ineffectiveness of medication due to poor technique | For Hitesh to be able to use his inhalers effectively | Teach Hitesh to breath in slowly and deeply while pressing the canister Record peak flow before and after bronchodilators |
| Potential lack of support on discharge | For Mr and Mrs Mahmoud to be aware of support services in the community | Give parents name and address of local and national asthma groups Inform health visitor and GP of admission and treatment Supply booklet for parents about asthma |

9.7 HEALTH EDUCATION

As well as the advice outlined previously, parents of children with chronic asthma need guidance about providing a relatively allergen-free environment. Those families who life in old, damp houses where there are increased numbers of dust mites should be classed as high priority for rehousing. Synthetic blankets, cotton sheets, foam pillows and mattresses, roller blinds and washable rugs are easier to keep dust- and mite-free. Daily damp dusting and vacuuming of carpets and upholstery when the child is out of the room reduces the incidence of mites. All rooms should be kept warm to inhibit damp and mould. A small bowl of water near the heat source will prevent the irritation of very dry heat. Tobacco smoke is another common irritant and smoking should not be allowed in the child's presence. Flowers should not be brought into the house as pollen is a potent allergen. Toys should be plastic, metal or wooden as these are easier to clean and keep dust free. As well as not always being washable, soft, stuffed toys can consist of irritant material. Foods known to precipitate attacks should be eliminated from the diet and food content labels should be read carefully to determine the presence of any known allergens.

Parents should also be helped to adopt a positive attitude towards their child's condition and to maintain a normal family life. Their behaviour towards the child should not alter and he should be allowed to participate, as far as he is able, in the normal activities of his age group. Liaison with playgroup or school will ensure that those involved in his care will be prepared for any problems. Parents and other carers should know what to do during an attack so that the chance of complications occurring is minimized. They should stay with the child and remain calm. He should be supported in a sitting position and allowed to rest. He should use his bronchodilator and hot drinks can be given to liquefy any secretions. The general practitioner should be contacted if the attack is severe and/or prolonged.

# 10 Care of the school-age child with epiglottitis

Epiglottitis is a bacterial infection which involves the soft tissues around the entrance to the larynx. Inflammation of the epiglottis and aryepiglottic folds causes obstruction of the upper airway. The onset and course of the infection is sudden and, unless the appropriate diagnosis and management is equally rapid, the outcome may be fatal. Indeed, before the advent of techniques to establish artificial airways, epiglottitis was commonly fatal. Because of the rapid obstructive process urgent treatment is vital and many hospitals have strict protocols for the management of children with upper airway obstruction to ensure that a senior anaesthetist is contacted in case urgent intubation is necessary.

Because the onset and course of the condition is so rapid, the child and his parents are very frightened. Their fear is compounded by the necessity for intubation and admission to the intensive care unit. The parents may also feel guilty that they did not appreciate the severity of the illness and may blame themselves, or each other, for the child's condition. The nurse must be sensitive to the child's need for reassurance and the parents' need to voice their feelings.

## 10.1 AETIOLOGY

### Incidence

Epiglottitis is mainly a paediatric entity, usually affecting children aged 3–7 years. It may occur in younger children but is rarely seen in those under 6 months or in adults. It occurs throughout the year with little seasonal variation.

## Causative organism

Most cases of epiglottitis are caused by the bacteria, *Haemophilus influenzae*, type B. Occasionally beta-haemolytic streptococci have been cultured and, rarely, staphylococci have been the cause of the condition.

## Transmission

Epiglottitis is usually preceded by a 24–48 h history of a minor upper respiratory tract infection. In young children the tip of the epiglottitis lies opposite the first cervical vertebra and spread of infection from other upper respiratory tract organs is relatively easy. Nursery and primary-school age children are particularly at risk of contracting droplet infections affecting the upper respiratory tract. Although the original infection may be transmitted to others by droplets the localization of the infection is individual to the affected child.

## 10.2 PATHOPHYSIOLOGY

The epiglottis is a leaf-shaped cartilage attached to the inner surface of the anterior wall of the thyroid cartilage. It acts like a lid over the entrance to the larynx. During the muscular action of swallowing the larynx moves upwards and forwards so that its opening is covered by the epiglottis allowing food and fluid to enter the oesophagus and not the airways. In the child the larynx lies approximately opposite the second, third and fourth cervical vertebra.

Once the bacterial infection of the epiglottis has become established the inflammatory response is provoked. The epiglottis becomes red, painful and grossly swollen (Figure 10.1) and its consequent loss of function inhibits swallowing. Inspiration while the epiglottis is swollen and occluding the larynx exaggerates the usual negative transpulmonary pressure present during this stage of respiration. The pressure may increase to a level where the lymphatics are no longer able to remove fluid from the alveolar capillaries. Perfusion of the alveoli is reduced and hypoxia results. Arteriolar constriction occurs as the body endeavours to improve alveolar perfusion which further increases pulmonary pressure. This rise in pressure leads to the formation of alveolar interstitial oedema.

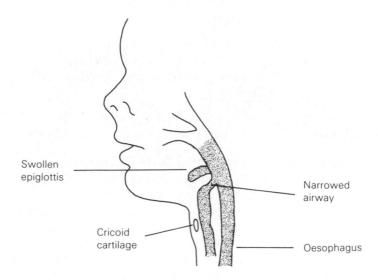

Swollen epiglottis

Narrowed airway

Cricoid cartilage

Oesophagus

**Figure 10.1**  Epiglottitis.

The highly negative interpleural pressure is also transmitted to the left ventricle and left ventricular output may decrease.

Spread of the initial infection results in a 25% incidence of pneumonia and cervical lymphadenitis. Otitis media may also result if the infection spreads via the eustachian tubes. The infection rarely spreads outside the respiratory tract although septicaemia can be a common complication.

Eventually the inflamed, swollen epiglottis will completely occlude the larynx and totally obstruct the airway. However, this event can be precipitated if the child is positioned in such a way that the larynx moves against the epiglottis, as occurs in swallowing. The two events which commonly precipitate asphyxia in this way are examination of the pharynx to visualize the epiglottis, and placing the child supine for investigation or treatment.

10.3 CLINICAL FEATURES

The parents of the child with epiglottitis usually report that the child had mild symptoms of a common cold which suddenly became much worse. Within about 4–6 h the child becomes pyrexial (38–40°C) and complains of a sore throat and of generally feeling unwell. During the next 2–4 h these features rapidly progress to severe dysphagia, the child being unable to swallow even saliva. As a result he refuses to eat or drink, and drooling of saliva occurs. Difficulty in breathing progresses to severe respiratory distress and the child begins to mouth breath. He adopts an upright position, leaning forward with his chin thrust out, to facilitate chest movements. Although chest retractions may be visible there is no obvious struggle to breathe as slow, quiet breathing allows better gaseous exchange. There is a croaking sound on inspiration and a snoring expiratory sound as air is forced through the narrow glottis. Due to the involvement of the vocal cords, the voice is thick and muffled. The child is pale or grey in colour and is obviously anxious and frightened by his condition. Late features, which occur when the obstruction has lead to hypoxia, are listlessness, cyanosis, and decreased sounds during inspiration and expiration.

Pharyngeal examination will reveal a red, inflamed throat and a distinctive large, cherry-red oedenatous epiglottis can be seen at the base of the tongue. However, this examination is only performed by an expert anaesthetist with intubation equipment, oxygen and suction available because of the danger of precipitating asphyxia.

## 10.4 INVESTIGATIONS

The clinical features and rapid progression of epiglottitis are so characteristic that the diagnosis is usually made from the appearance of the child and the history of his illness from his parents. To confirm the diagnosis lateral neck X-rays can be taken. These will reveal a thumb-shaped thickening of the epiglottic and supraglottic swelling. Approximately 50–70% of affected children will have positive blood cultures and once intubation has been performed, tracheal secretions and/or swabs of the epiglottis can be sent to the laboratory for microscopy, culture and sensitivity. This will ensure that the causative organism is sensitive to the chosen antibiotic therapy.

If pulmonary oedema is present, specimens of arterial blood should be obtained to ascertain blood gases and pH.

## 10.5 MEDICAL MANAGEMENT

Epiglottitis requires immediate relief of the obstruction to prevent total occlusion of the airway. Epiglottic swelling usually alters the anatomy of the glottis and therefore intubation is usually performed in the operating theatre. The child remains in the sitting position and is anaesthetized with the use of an inhalation agent and oxygen. Muscle relaxants are not used when the airway is severely compromised as they may precipitate asphyxia. An endotracheal tube, one size smaller than usual to allow for the laryngeal swelling, is initially used to provide a clear airway. The size of the tube usually used for intubating children over 2 years is estimated as follows:

$$\text{Endotracheal tube size} = \frac{\text{Age in years}}{4} + 4.5$$

Once the obstruction has been bypassed by this procedure, a nasotracheal tube can be put into position. If necessary, confirmation of the diagnosis by visual examination and culture of the epiglottis can be done at this time. A further X-ray of the neck and chest will confirm the correct position of the nasotracheal tube and will reveal the presence of any pulmonary infiltrates and oedema. Humidified oxygen is given via the nasotracheal tube and continuous positive airway pressure and mechanical ventilation may be necessary to stabilize blood gases. Chest physiotherapy should be performed 4 hourly to prevent atelectasis. Intubation usually results in a marked improvement but extubation is not usually considered until the child has received at least 24 h of intravenous antibiotic therapy. A 10-day course of antibiotics is commenced. Ampicillin 150 mg/kg/day and chloramphenical 50–75 mg/kg/day are usually given until the laboratory confirms the causative organism and its sensitivity. Antipyretics may be necessary if the child's temperature rises to about 38.5°C.

An intravenous infusion is commenced to maintain hydration until the child can swallow again. Once swallowing is possible, the child is apyrexial and the inflammation of the epiglottis has resolved, the child can be extubated. This usually occurs 36–48 h after admission.

10.6 NURSING CARE

**Assessment**

*Breathing*

- What is the child's respiratory rate?
- What colour is the child?
- Are chest retractions visible?
- Is he mouth-breathing?
- Are respirations noisy?

*Maintaining body temperature*

- What is the child's temperature?

*Eating and drinking*

- Is the child able to swallow?
- Is the child drooling?
- Has the child been eating and drinking at home?

*Rest and sleep*

- What position does the child adopt as the most comfortable?

*Communication*

- What does the child's speech sound like?

**Planning**

Nursing care of the child with epiglottitis is primarily concerned with ensuring that the child maintains a clear airway. Until the child is intubated he should be nursed in the upright position and never in the horizontal position. The nurse should stay with the child and observe him continuously for any signs of deterioration, such as:

- marked progressive restlessness and anxiety;
- cyanosis;
- marked suprasternal and intercostal retractions;
- decreasing respiratory rate;
- increasing pyrexia and tachycardia.

**Table 10.1** Care plan for the schoolchild with epiglottitis. Benjamin Seigler, aged 7 years, has been admitted to the intensive care unit. He arrived in casualty an hour ago in severe respiratory distress with a hyperpyrexia of 40°C and drooling. His parents reported that they had kept him away from school with a sore throat and mild temperature for 24 h but that he had suddenly become much worse. Once seen by the paediatrician a diagnosis of epiglottitis was made and he was transferred to theatre for intubation. Lateral neck X-rays performed in theatre confirmed the diagnosis. Blood and hypopharyngeal cultures were also performed in theatre

| Problem | Aim of care | Nursing intervention |
| --- | --- | --- |
| Potential asphyxia due to accidental movement of nasotracheal tube | For Ben's nasotracheal tube to remain in the correct position | Observe Ben continuously for signs of dislodged tube (sudden cyanosis, audible cry, chest retractions) <br> Ensure tube tapes are always secure <br> Ensure Ben cannot reach tube. Use arm splints if necessary <br> Give prescribed sedation if Ben is very restless |
| Potential asphyxia due to obstruction of Ben's nasotracheal tube | For Ben's nasotracheal tube to remain patent | Observe Ben for signs of obstruction (cyanosis, laboured, noisy breathing, tachycardia) <br> Apply suction hourly after instillation of 0.5 ml normal saline into tube. Perform more frequently if secretions thick <br> Administer humidified 40% oxygen |
| Ben is unable to swallow due to sore and swollen throat | To handle Ben's secretions and provide him with IV fluids until he can swallow | Suction mouth gently as necessary <br> Position Ben upright or laterally <br> Do not give oral fluids <br> Ensure parenteral fluids are running at the prescribed rate |

| | | |
|---|---|---|
| Ben is unable to rest due to fear of his strange environment and treatment | For Ben to look relaxed and be able to rest | Reassure Ben repeatedly that the tube will be removed as soon as he is better<br>Explain all procedures and his surroundings<br>Nurse or parents to cuddle him on lap if very anxious |
| Pyrexia | For Ben's temperature to be within normal limits in 24 h | Provide light clothing and bedding<br>Use fan to cool environment (do not direct at child)<br>Administer prescribed anti-pyretic<br>Monitor axilla temperature hourly<br>Administer prescribed antibiotics |
| Parental anxiety due to Ben's sudden severe illness | To encourage Mr and Mrs Seigler to share their concerns and ask questions | Give parents opportunity to talk and ask questions<br>Explain usual course of events<br>Explain all procedures<br>Allow them to participate in Ben's care |

Low concentrations of humidified oxygen should be given and resuscitation equipment should be readily available. X-rays are best performed on the ward in the presence of intubation equipment.

After intubation the child should continue to be closely observed for any signs of increasing obstruction or further complications. Arm restraints or sedation may be necessary as the child soon feels better and may try to pull his nasotracheal tube out. Oxygen should continue with 2–4 hourly suction and chest physiotherapy to remove secretions and prevent pneumonia atelectasis.

If the child has a pyrexia of 38.5°C or above, cooling measures should be employed and an antipyretic such as Calpol given at 4 hourly intervals. The pyrexia usually responds quickly to antibiotic therapy and usually returns to normal within 48 h.

The rapid progression of epiglottitis and the child's frightening appearance finishing with his admission to an intensive care unit is an alarming experience for the parents. They may also feel guilty for not having realized the seriousness or urgency of their child's condition. The nurse should recognize that these feelings may possibly be present.

If sedation has been given, the effects of this should be allowed to wear off before extubation. After removal of the nasotracheal tube the child should remain in the intensive care unit under close observation for 3–4 h in case there is any recurrence of obstruction. Once this time has passed with no problems and the child is taking oral fluids, he can be transferred to a unit of lesser dependency. The child is ready for discharge when he is apyrexial and able to take his usual diet, usually after a further 48–72 h. Parents should be given clear instructions to ensure the child completes his course of antibiotics. The care plan of a child with epiglottitis is shown in Table 10.1.


10.7 HEALTH EDUCATION

When a child is discharged in the middle of a course of antibiotics it is important that his parents understand the importance of antibiotic therapy. The nurse should explain the following:

- Antibiotics are chemical substances which have the capacity to kill or inhibit the growth of bacteria.
- Although the child is much better, the bottle of elixir or capsules should be finished. To stop before the full amount has been taken can lead to a recurrence of the infection.
- Some diarrhoea may be experienced as antibiotics can destroy the bacteria that normally inhibit the bowel. Profuse diarrhoea and/or vomiting should be reported to the general practitioner as the drug will no longer be absorbed or effective.
- The antibiotics should be taken in the amount and frequency advised on the bottle. Too much may cause diarrhoea, too little will destroy its effectiveness.
- To ensure a constant level of antibiotics in the blood-stream, the elixir or capsules should be given at regular intervals throughout each 24 h as far as possible.

# 11 Care of the older child with pneumonia

Pneumonia is a general term used to describe an acute inflammation of the pulmonary parenchyma. It is usually caused by an infective agent but it can also be due to physical, chemical or allergic factors. Pneumonias can be classified in three ways, according to clinical form, morphology or aetiology. Clinically, pneumonia may occur as a primary disease or it may be secondary to debilitating conditions such as whooping cough or measles. Morphologically, pneumonias can be subdivided into three main types. Lobar pneumonia, which is rarely seen nowadays, is inflammation of a large segment of one or more lobes of the lung. This type of pneumonia may affect only one lung or be bilateral. (Bilateral lobar pneumonia used to be termed 'double pneumonia'.) Bronchopneumonia begins in the terminal bronchioles and becomes widespread involving much of the pulmonary parenchyma in the base of the lung. In interstitial pneumonia the inflammation is mainly confined within the walls of the alveoli. The most useful classification of pneumonia is by aetiology. There are four main causes of pneumonia: bacteria, viruses, myoplasms and aspiration of physical, chemical or allergic substances.

## 11.1 AETIOLOGY

### Incidence

Primary infective pneumonia generally occurs most often during the spring and autumn months. Secondary infective pneumonia is more prevalent during the winter when other respiratory infections are at their peak. Secondary infective

**Table 11.1** Incidence of infective pnemonias

| Type of pneumonia | Commonest age group affected | Seasonal variation | Other factors |
|---|---|---|---|
| Pneumococcal | 1–4 years | Feb–March | Commonest cause of acute pneumonia |
| Staphylococcal | 1–2 years | Dec–Feb | Can be a hospital-acquired infection |
| Streptococcal | 1–5 years | Jan–March | Often complicates influenza A or measles |
| Viral pneumonia | All ages | – | Often associated with other viral upper respiratory infections |
| Mycoplasmal pneumonia | 1–4 years | Sept–Dec | Occurs more often in crowded living conditions |

pneumonia is sometimes seen in epidemics in association with widespread outbreaks of influenza. Other factors influencing the incidence of infective pneumonia are related to the specific causative organism (Table 11.1).

Pneumonia which occurs as the result of irritation from foreign material is common amongst children. The newborn may develop pneumonia during birth from the aspiration of amniotic fluid and other debris. The infant is liable to aspirate food or secretions if placed on his back after feeding, or he can develop aspiration pneumonia from the inhalation of vigorously used talcum powder. A child who is weak or paralysed or has a congenital problem which interferes with feeding, such as cleft palate, trache-oesophageal fistula or hiatus hernia, is also liable to aspirate food or secretions due to his inability or difficulty in swallowing. Aspiration of foreign bodies can occur at any age but it is commonest in the child who is between 1 and 3 years who, characteristically, explores everything with his mouth. Near drowning, or survival after submersion in a fluid medium, can also be a cause of aspiration pneumonia in children under 3 years of age but the majority of these situations involve children between 10 and 16 years.

### Causative organisms

There are many infective agents which cause pneumonia during childhood (Figure 11.1). Their prevalence depends on the age of the child and the child's general state of health at the time of infection. Some infective agents only cause pneumonia when the child's immune response is depressed. These agents or opportunistic organisms are otherwise incapable of causing respiratory infection. A common example is cytomegalovirus which can cause pneumonia in children who have been receiving large doses of corticosteroids or immunosuppressive drugs after transplantation or during treatment for leukaemia. Pneumonia which occurs following aspiration of fluids, food or vomit may be caused by *Pseudomonas aeruginosa, Escherichia coli* or anaerobic organisms contained within the aspirate. Alternatively, the inflammation may simply be the response to the presence of the foreign material. This latter cause of pneumonia can also result from the inhalation of poisonous gases (chemical pneumonia), a chest injury which disturbs normal respiration (traumatic pneumonia) or inhalation of oily substances such as liquid paraffin (lipoid pneumonia).

### Transmission

Pathogenic organisms can reach the lungs in four ways. Inhalation of organisms suspended in the air (droplet infection) is the commonest route of infection for viral respiratory infections. Bacteria are usually carried to the lungs by aspiration of oropharyngeal secretions. Ingestion of chemical substances usually causes coughing and vomiting which results in aspiration of the substance which then gives rise to parenchymal inflammation.

The circulatory system can carry viruses and bacteria to the lungs from primary infection sites, such as the heart, urinary tract or the skin of children with burns. Rarely, direct contact can spread infection to the lungs via a subphrenic abscess or a penetrating chest wound.

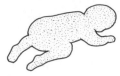

**Previously healthy infants**
Respiratory syncytial virus
Adenovirus
Bacteria

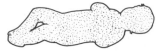

**Unwell, debilitated infants**
*Staphylococcus*
*E. coli*
Viruses and opportunistic organisms

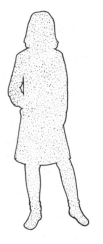

**Children 1–16 years**
Virus
*Pneumococcus*
Mycoplasma

**Figure 11.1** The common organisms causing pneumonia in childhood.

## 11.2 PATHOPHYSIOLOGY

The normal body defences against infection entering the lungs are usually so efficient that pneumonia usually only occurs when the body is already weakened or when there are overwhelming noxious stimuli.

Various factors can adversely affect the body's natural defence mechanisms and allow parenchymal infection to occur. The child who has a decreased level of consciousness due to drugs, neurological disorders or head injury has impaired cough and gag reflexes which predisposes him to aspiration of food, fluid or secretions. Long-term use of nasogastric, naso-endotracheal and endotracheal tubes can also impair the cough and gag reflexes.

The child who usually mouth-breathes inspires poorly humidified air because the nasal cilia have been bypassed. As a consequence the cilia become brittle and the mucus thick and tenacious, predisposing to infection. Chronic mouth breathing can be seen in children with chronic respiratory disorders, such as cystic fibrosis, and those with a chronic obstruction such as that caused by chronically infected adenoids.

Hypoventilation of lung tissue, which can occur if a child lies still in bed breathing with only a part of his lung due to pain or immobility, can cause stasis of bronchial secretions and predispose to infection.

Environmental pollution, such as that which occurs in the home when both parents are heavy smokers, may compromise macrophage function and allow parenchymal infection to occur.

Once bacteria reach the alveoli they act as irritants. The alveoli become inflamed and oedematous. The alveolar capillaries become swollen with blood and increased numbers of white cells. Eventually this blood and exudate passes into the alveoli where it acts as an ideal culture medium. As the bacteria multiply, the inflammatory response increases and more fluid enters the alveoli and the pneumonia spreads. As the affected child breathes and coughs more alveoli and the bronchioles become involved.

Viruses usually first attack the epithelial cells of the bronchioles. Interstitial inflammation and desquamation result and rapidly spread to involve the alveoli which fill with exudate.

Aspiration of gastric juices or chemicals usually involves the right lung because the right bronchus lies more in line with the trachea. The aspirate may cause direct damage to the respiratory mucosa. The inflammation which results causes pulmonary oedema and the alveoli fill with exudate. Particles within the aspirate may also obstruct the smaller airways causing stasis of secretions distal to the blockage and predisposing to secondary bacterial infection. A pocket of infection around the aspirated foreign matter can lead to abscess formation.

Whatever the primary cause of the inflammation, once the alveoli are full of exudate (consolidated), gaseous exchange is impossible and hypoxia occurs. The inflamed lung tissue may also infect the surrounding pleura and spread to involve the rest of the respiratory tract. The mucous membranes of the nose, pharynx, trachea and bronchi become inflamed and the collection of exudate in these airways causes coughing and expectoration. As the inflammation continues, blood from the swollen mucosa colours the sputum a rusty red.

## 11.3 CLINICAL FEATURES

The clinical features of pneumonia vary according to its cause (Table 11.2). Apart from in the bacterial types, the infection commences gradually with systemic features. The specific features of parenchymal infection follow within 6–36 h. Nowadays these later characteristic signs of pneumonia are rarely seen due to prompt and efficient treatment. However, many infants and small children with little or no immunity to bacterial infection, develop complications such as empyema or pyopneumothorax, as a result of staphylococcal pneumonia. Nonpurulent effusions may complicate pneumococcal pneumonia.

## 11.4 INVESTIGATIONS

The diagnosis of pneumonia is usually made by the combination of the parents' history of the illness and the child's clinical features. A sputum specimen for microscopy, culture and sensitivity should be taken before antibiotic treatment is commenced. The choice of antibiotic used depends on a positive identification of the causative organism. In severely ill children a blood culture may also be performed. A chest X-ray may help to identify the organism by revealing the extent and pattern of the infection. Consolidation of a lobe of one lung is characteristic of pneumococcal pneumonia and staphylococcal pneumonia always produces multiple pulmonary abscesses. Viral pneumonia is confirmed by diffuse areas of patchy infiltration of the bronchioles. A diagnosis of staphylococcal pneumonia is further confirmed by a marked leucocytosis. In myoplasmal pneumonia the white cell count is often normal or below normal.

**Table 11.2** Comparative and contrasting features of different types of pneumonia

| Characteristics | Bacterial pneumonia | Viral pneumonia | Mycoplasmal pneumonia | Aspiration pneumonia |
|---|---|---|---|---|
| Onset | Sudden | Gradual | Sudden or insiduous | Gradual. Usually 24–48 h after aspiration |
| Initial features | Pyrexia and tachycardia. Rapid, shallow respirations. Productive cough (purulent rusty sputum). Restlessness, apprehension. Chest pain (may be referred to abdomen in young children) | Mild fever. Slight cough (unproductive or productive of small amounts of white sputum). General malaise | Pyrexia. Non-productive cough. General malaise | No pyrexia. Productive cough (white sputum possibly containing foreign matter) |
| Later features | Rapid progression of symptoms: Meningism Drowsiness Respiratory distress | Hyperpyrexia, dyspnoea and cyanosis. Productive cough (copious amounts of blood-streaked sputum) | Productive cough (sero-mucoid – mucopurulent and blood streaked) | Pyrexia. Dyspnoea. Haemoptysis |

If the history reveals the possibility of foreign body aspiration a bronchoscopy is usually performed. X-rays will show the position of opaque foreign bodies but are of little use if the aspirate consists of vegetable matter. The bronchoscopy should be performed as soon as possible before the inflammatory process makes removal of the foreign body too difficult.

## 11.5 MEDICAL MANAGEMENT

Not all children with pneumonia require admission to hospital. Most older children with pneumococcal pneumonia can be nursed at home. Hospitalization is usually only recommended for infants, for children with staphylococcal pneumonia and those with complications such as pleural effusion of empyema.

Children who require treatment in hospital usually need supplemental humidified oxygen to reduce the restlessness caused by hypoxia. Intravenous fluids replace fluids lost by tachypnoea and overcomes the infant's inability to suck when breathless. An antipyretic will prevent febrile convulsions in the under-5s and also provide relief of chest and muscle pain. The choice of antibiotic will depend on the causative organism but occasionally organisms have proved resistant and a combination of drugs is usually prescribed as follows:

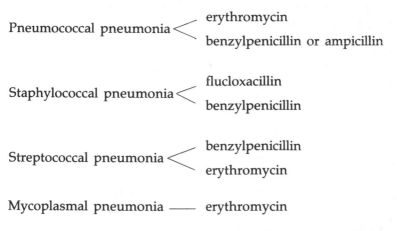

Pneumococcal pneumonia
- erythromycin
- benzylpenicillin or ampicillin

Staphylococcal pneumonia
- flucloxacillin
- benzylpenicillin

Streptococcal pneumonia
- benzylpenicillin
- erythromycin

Mycoplasmal pneumonia —— erythromycin

Antibiotics are usually given parenterally initially and then orally until the 7–10 day course is complete. The child usually responds in 36–48 h becoming apyrexial and less breathless.

Occasionally prophylatic antibiotics may be given to children with viral pneumonia or to those with any type of aspiration pneumonia to reduce or prevent secondary bacterial infection.

If pleural effusion is present a diagnostic aspiration of the chest is usually performed. Continuous closed chest drainage is instituted if purulent fluid is withdrawn, a common finding in children with staphylococcal pneumonia.

The prognosis and course of pneumonia varies according to the causative organism and the speed of diagnosis and treatment. Most types of pneumonia have a good prognosis although the resolution of the infection may take from 1 to 6 weeks depending on the age and general health of the child. Staphylococcal pneumonia is the most serious form of infection and has a mortality rate of about 20%.

## 11.6 NURSING CARE

### Assessment

### *Breathing*

- What is the child's pulse and respiratory rate?
- Does he show any signs of dyspnoea? What signs are these?
- Does the child have a cough? Is it productive?
- If the cough is productive how much expectorate is produced? What does this expectorate look like?
- What is the child's colour?

### *Maintaining body temperature*

- What is the child's temperature?
- Does his skin feel hot and dry or cold and clammy?

### *Eating and drinking*

- Has the child lost his normal appetite?
- Has breathlessness interfered with the child's usual eating and drinking? What can he manage to eat and drink?

### *Rest and sleep*

- Has pain interfered with this? Where is the pain? What makes it better or worse?

• Is the child lethargic or restless?

## Communication

• Does breathlessness and/or pain make this difficult?
• Does the child appear anxious?

## Maintaining a safe environment

• Has the child shown any signs of a mild upper respiratory infection within the last 24–72 h or has there been any recent vomiting or choking which may have caused an aspiration pneumonia?

## Planning

The nursing care of a child with pneumonia is mainly symptomatic and supportive. The child at home can be nursed in bed, given prescribed antipyretics and antibiotics, and encouraged to drink liberal amounts of 'clear' fluids. The child in·hospital has more severe features but these main principles of care remain the same (Table 11.3). Breathlessness can be relieved by rest, an upright position and the administration of humidified oxygen. The cool temperature of the humidified oxygen also helps to reduce the child's pyrexia. Careful handling and positioning the child on his affected side helps to relieve pain. Support for the affected side of the chest decreases the discomfort of pleural rubbing.

Vital signs must be recorded at regular intervals to monitor the course of the condition and to facilitate the early detection of complications. A rapid rise in temperature may precede a febrile convulsion in the young child. An increased pulse and respiratory rate and restlessness indicate hypoxia. Later features of hypoxia are cyanosis and a decreased level of consciousness. Any expectorate should also be observed carefully. Blood-streaked purulent sputum of increased viscosity indicates deterioration. Earache or pain around the sinuses may indicate spread of the infection and the presence of otitis media or sinusitis.

Young children or those who are too ill to expectorate may need suctioning to maintain a patent airway. All children may benefit from percussion and vibration prior to suctioning, or

**Table 11.3** Care plan for a schoolchild with pneumonia. Ian Jones, aged 10, has been admitted from home with pneumonia. He has been ill at home for 3 days with no response to oral antibiotic treatment. On admission he looks feverish and breathless, and has a temperature of 40°C, a tachycardia of 100 and a respiratory rate of 30. He has a productive cough but is having difficulty expectorating due to right-sided chest pain. Ian lives with his father who is unable to take time off work to stay with him

| Problem | Aim of care | Nursing intervention |
|---|---|---|
| Dyspnoea (respiratory rate = 30) and tachycardia (pulse = 100) due to hypoxia | To improve Ian's oxygenation so that he is able to breathe without difficulty at a rate of 16–20/min and have a decreased pulse rate | Nurse Ian at rest and help him with all activities of living<br>Position Ian in the orthopnoeic position<br>Administer humidified oxygen via nasal cannulae<br>Observe and record Ian's respiratory rate and effort, and pulse hourly |
| Pyrexia (40°C) due to infection | For Ian's temperature to return to normal limits | Administer prescribed IV antibiotics<br>Administer prescribed antipyretics 4 hourly while pyrexial<br>Record Ian's temperature hourly<br>Nurse Ian with minimal bedcovers<br>Provide a fan by his bed |
| Ian is restless and uncomfortable due to right-sided chest pain and fear | To help Ian to rest in comfort | Position Ian on his right side<br>Administer prescribed analgesics 4 hourly<br>Observe and question Ian about the effect of pain relieving measures<br>Plan Ian's care to avoid excessive movement and allow rest<br>Explain all care |

| Problem | Goal | Nursing action |
|---|---|---|
| Productive cough due to excessive secretions | To help Ian to expectorate | Chest physiotherapy – to encourage Ian to cough<br>Encourage Ian to drink about 200 ml at hourly intervals (he likes coke, lemon squash and milky tea)<br>Relieve pain as above<br>Provide sputum pot and tissues in easy reach |
| Potential spread of infection causing otitis media, sinusitis, lung abscess | To observe Ian for any features of deterioration | Observe Ian for earache or headache<br>Observe the amount, colour and character of Ian's sputum. Report any changes |
| Potential dehydration due to increased fluid loss and anorexia | To ensure Ian has a positive fluid balance | Encourage oral fluids as above<br>Record all intake and output |
| Potential pressure sores due to immobility | To ensure Ian's skin remains intact and healthy | Encourage Ian to change his position 2 hourly<br>If Ian is sweaty, wash and dry skin<br>Observe all pressure areas for redness during bed bath |
| Potential constipation due to pyrexia, antipyretics and immobility | To help Ian maintain his normal elimination routine. (Bowels open daily after breakfast) | Offer bedpan after breakfast<br>Encourage fresh fruit and fluids<br>Record when Ian has his bowels open |

**Table 11.3** contd

| Problem | Aim of care | Nursing intervention |
|---|---|---|
| Potential clotting problems due to immobility | To help Ian exercise to promote venous return | Encourage deep breathing and leg exercises<br>Ensure 2 hourly change of position as above<br>Observe Ian for any complaints of:<br>  generalized chest pain<br>  calf pain |
| Potential anxiety due to Ian's separation from his family, peers and daily activities | For Ian to feel safe and at ease in hospital | Provide continuity of care<br>Stay with Ian as much as possible<br>Allow Ian to express his concerns<br>Explain honestly all care<br>Encourage Ian's family to visit or 'phone when they are able<br>Keep to Ian's normal routine for activities of daily living |
| Ian is unable to attend to his own personal hygiene due to breathlessness and malaise | For Ian to have help with washing and dressing until he feels able to do this independently | Wash Ian in bed daily<br>Help Ian to brush his teeth and hair<br>Offer mouthwashes<br>Offer bowl for handwashing after use of bottle and bedpan |

postural drainage to help the expectoration of secretions. The presence of sputum together with mouth-breathing causes a dry and dirty mouth. Mouth care will help to ease this discomfort if the child is too ill to take oral fluids.

Children with a staphylococcal infection are usually the most seriously affected and are isolated to prevent cross infection. Apart from these individuals and those whose pneumonia is secondary to other illnesses, children with pneumonia usually recover quickly.

## 11.7 HEALTH EDUCATION

Aspiration pneumonia can be prevented. At birth a mucus trap should be used to clear the neonate's pharynx and nasal passages and prevent aspiration of amniotic fluid and mucus. Mothers should be shown how to position their baby on his right side or abdomen after feeding to prevent aspiration. His clothing and bedlinen should be loose enough to allow him full lung expansion. During bathing any crusting of his nostrils should be cleared and ideally talcum powder should not be used as this light powder is easily inhaled.

Solid foods should not be introduced into a child's diet until he is about 1 year old and can chew properly. At this age his food should be cut into bite-size pieces and he should be taught not to talk while eating. Proper feeding techniques should be carried out for handicapped or debilitated children. Uncooperative children should never be force fed. Children under 3 years of age should not be allowed to eat nuts or popcorn on which they may choke. Also, they should not be allowed to play with small objects which may be put in the mouth. Coins, nails, screws, safety pins, buttons and other small household objects should be kept out of the child's reach. These young children should always be supervised when near water because of the danger of falling. Older children should be taught the danger of water if they cannot swim. All parents should know how to deal effectively with a child who is choking (Figures 11.2–11.4).

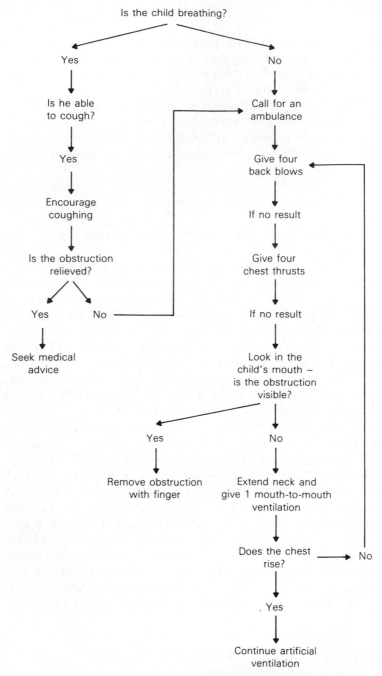

**Figure 11.2** Advice for parents on how to deal with a choking infant or child.

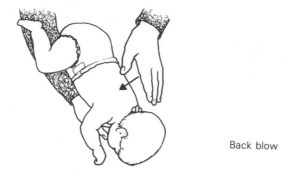

Back blow

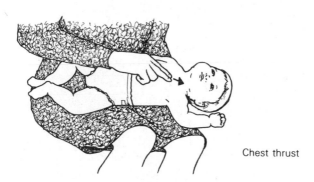

Chest thrust

**Figure 11.3** Management of a choking infant.

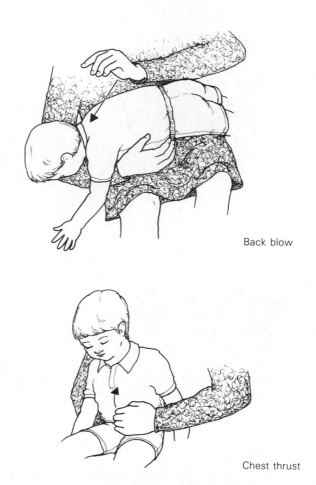

Back blow

Chest thrust

**Figure 11.4** Management of a choking child.

# 12 Care of the adolescent with cystic fibrosis

Cystic fibrosis is an inherited condition which affects the exocrine glands. The lungs and the pancreas are the organs primarily involved. It is the most common and one of the most serious genetic disorders in the United Kingdom. It was first recognized in the 1930s when 90% of affected children died within the first year of life. Although cystic fibrosis can still be fatal, improvements in treatment have resulted in a steady increase in life expectancy. At present, 65% of affected children in England and Wales will survive until adulthood (18 years). The median age of survival has risen from 2 years in 1940 to approximately 30 years. The quality of life for those affected has also improved with at least 75% of adults with cystic fibrosis beng active and in full-time employment.

Although the prognosis in cystic fibrosis has greatly improved, the condition can cause considerable upheaval for the child and his family. The modification of numerous family activities and the responsibility of caring for a chronically ill child can tax family relationships. The nurse needs to be alert to these stresses and be able to offer psychological support as well as nursing care to the child and his family.

## 12.1 AETIOLOGY

### Incidence

The prevalence of cystic fibrosis in Europeans is approximately 1 in 2500. It is more common in central Europeans and occurs in 1 in 1600 children in the United Kingdom resulting in about 450 new cases per year. It is much less common outside

Europe, the reason for this disparity is at present unknown. Only 1 in 17 000 negroids and 1 in 90 000 orientals are affected. Boys and girls are equally affected.

### Causative factors

The basic defect which causes the various clinical features of cystic fibrosis is currently unknown. Recent research seems to indicate that a defect in chloride transport may be the single abnormality which causes the widespread manifestations of cystic fibrosis. It appears that the features of cystic fibrosis may all be due to an inhibition in the reabsorption of chloride across the gland ducts. A decrease in chloride ion permeability has been found in the sweat glands, respiratory epithelium and placental membranes of babies with cystic fibrosis.

### Transmission

Cystic fibrosis is inherited as an autosomal recessive trait. In the United Kingdom 1 in 25 people carry the gene for the disease but because it is a recessive gene they are unaffected. However, when two of these apparently normal people have children, there is a 25% chance that any such children will receive one abnormal gene from each of them and develop cystic fibrosis (Figure 12.1).

Recent research, using recombinant DNA techniques, has identified the short arm of chromosome numer 7 as the site of the faulty gene. Further study is now concentrating on discovering which of the genes on this chromosome is defective. The identification of the specific defective gene will make it possible to identify carriers, permit genetic counselling of carriers and to identify affected fetuses, and offer therapeutic abortion if necessary.

At present there is no reliable means of identifying carriers of cystic fibrosis. Amniocentesis may reveal a marked decrease in the intestinal isoenzyme alkaline phosphatase. This test, which is probably only 70% reliable, is offered only to parents who already have a child with cystic fibrosis and thus are known carriers.

The vast majority of males with cystic fibrosis are sterile and affected females have a low fertility. If a cystic fibrosis woman has a partner who carries the cystic fibrosis gene, each of their

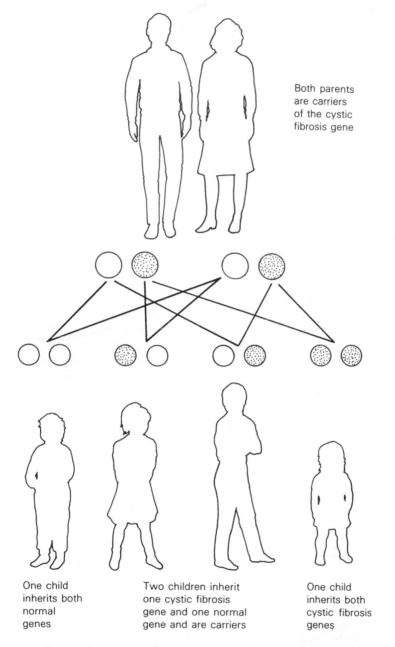

Both parents
are carriers
of the cystic
fibrosis gene

One child
inherits both
normal
genes

Two children inherit
one cystic fibrosis
gene and one normal
gene and are carriers

One child
inherits both
cystic fibrosis
genes

**Figure 12.1** Mode of inheritance of cystic fibrosis where both parents are carriers.

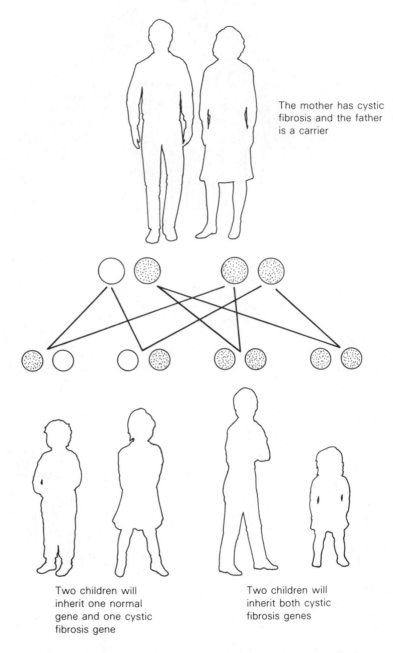

The mother has cystic fibrosis and the father is a carrier

Two children will inherit one normal gene and one cystic fibrosis gene

Two children will inherit both cystic fibrosis genes

**Figure 12.2** Mode of inheritance of cystic fibrosis where the woman has the disease and the man is a carrier.

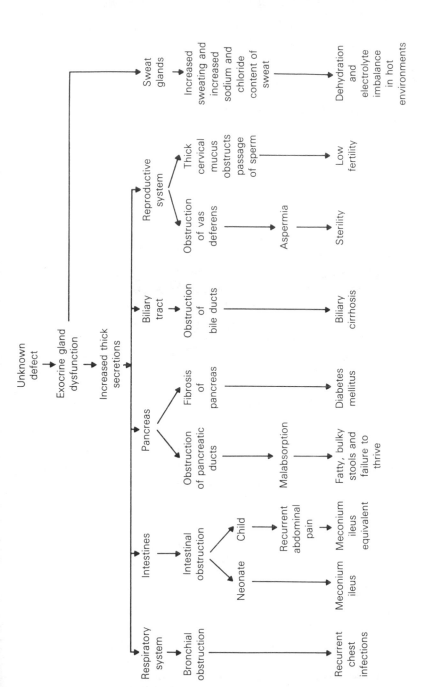

**Figure 12.3** The pathophysiology of cystic fibrosis.

children would have a 50% chance of inheriting the mother's condition (Figure 12.2).

## 12.2 PATHOPHYSIOLOGY

The unknown defect responsible for cystic fibrosis causes an increase in the viscosity of the secretions of the exocrine glands. Instead of producing thin, flowing secretions, the mucus-forming glands secrete a thick, sticky mucoprotein that precipitates or coagulates in the glands and ducts resulting in obstruction of the affected organ. Cystic fibrosis, therefore, affects multiple organ systems but the degree of dysfunction varies with each individual child (Figure 12.3).

Pulmonary dysfunction is present to some degree in almost all children with cystic fibrosis and is the main cause of death. Children with cystic fibrosis have normal lungs at birth but within a few months changes can be found. The abnormally thick and sticky mucus obstructs the bronchioles causing collapse of the alveoli distal to the obstruction and hyperinflation of the airways proximal to the obstruction. The retained mucus provides an ideal medium for the growth of bacteria. Serious pathogens such as *Staphylococcus aureus* and Pseudomonas aeruginosa are common to those with cystic fibrosis and the prognosis of the condition is probably related to the interaction between the affected child and the infecting organism.

Infection causes a localized suppurative bronchopneumonia and necrosis of lung tissue. Extensive bronchiectasis, bronchopneumonia and lung abscesses occur eventually leading to fibrosis and cyst formation.

As the pulmonary function progresses there is a gradual deterioration in vital capacity and gaseous exchange. Initially, increased muscularization of the pulmonary vessels occurs in an attempt to overcome the poor oxygenation. The right ventricle tries to force blood into the fibrosed lungs but eventually the pressure required is too great and cardiac failure ensues (Figure 12.4).

## 12.3 CLINICAL FEATURES

Children with cystic fibrosis present in different ways and at different ages according to the severity of their disease (Figure

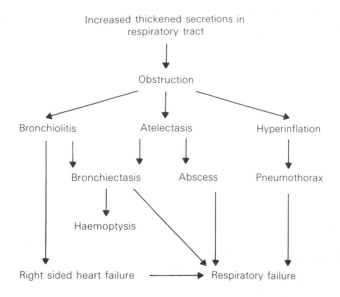

**Figure 12.4** The progression of lung dysfunction in cystic fibrosis.

12.5). Some children may present in infancy with severe respiratory infection which rapidly progresses to respiratory failure and death. Other children may not be diagnosed until adolescence during investigation for recurrent abdominal pain or for delay in sexual development.

The majority of children with cystic fibrosis present during early childhood and some degree of obstructive pulmonary disease with increased cough and sputum, finger clubbing and decreased respiratory function is the most common mode of presentation. For this reason cystic fibrosis should not be ruled out in any pre-school child who presents with:

- recurrent episodes of bronchiolitis;
- persistent wheeze and dyspnoea;
- persistent productive cough and clubbing;
- purulent sputum which cultures pseudomonas.

## 12.4 INVESTIGATIONS

The only certain diagnostic test for cystic fibrosis is the sweat test (Figure 12.6). This is only a reliable test when sodium or

Presentation in the neonate

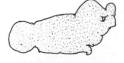

Meconium ileus
(10–15%)

Presentation in early infancy

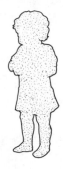

Respiratory
features
(40%)

{ Noisy and wheezing
breathing

Harsh cough

Recurrent chest
infections

Features of
malabsorption
(30%)

{ Fatty, bulky stools

Rectal prolapse

Slow weight gain

Excessive
sweating
(5%)

{ Salty taste when kissed

Rapid finger wrinkling
in water

Heat prostration or
dehydration in heat

**Figure 12.5** Features of cystic fibrosis at different ages.

Presentation in later childhood

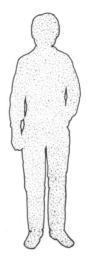

Later complications
(10%)
{
  *Cirrhosis*

  *Sinusitis*

  *Diabetes mellitus*

  *Delayed puberty*

  *Recurrent abdominal pain*
}

**Figure 12.5** contd

chloride level is over 60 mmol/l. The test is less accurate after puberty as some normal adolescents have sweat electrolyte values as high as 90 mmol/l. The sweat test is usually repeated if the result is inconclusive.

Two sweat sodium levels of over 70 mmol/l are considered diagnostic of cystic fibrosis. Because of the difficulty in determining the result of some tests it is important that the sweat test is performed by an expert technician in a specialist cystic fibrosis centre.

The standard sweat test is performed by pilocarpine ionophoresis. A small electric current is passed through a pilocarpine solution applied to the skin of the forearm. The local concentration of the drug stimulates the surrounding sweat

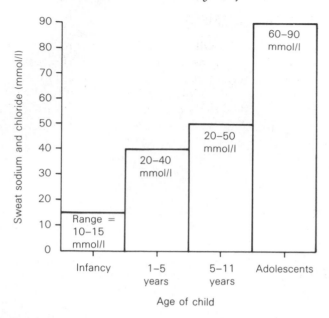

**Figure 12.6** The range of normal sweat electrolyte values.

glands. A dry pre-weighed filter paper is placed on the ionto-phoresed area of skin and made airtight with polythene. A bandage holds this in place and added clothing enhances sweating. After about 20 min the filter paper is removed for laboratory testing.

If the result of the sweat test is inconclusive other tests may aid the diagnosis. A 3-day collection of stools for fat estimation may reveal steatorrhoea which is present in most children with cystic fibrosis. Pancreatic enzyme tests are abnormal in most cystic fibrosis children. After a 6-hour fast a nasoduodenal tube is passed, and collections of fasting juices taken. Further timed specimens are collected after an intravenous injection of pancreozymin-cholecystokinin. The laboratory can then analyse the specimens for trypsin, lipase and pancreatic amylase. Pancreatic enzyme tests can also be carried out on stools.

It is technically possible to screen all neonates for cystic fibrosis by measuring the serium immunoreactive trypsin which is markedly increased in the newborn with cystic fibrosis. This is presently a very controversial issue as the cost of such a test is approximately £800 for each positively diagnosed neonate.

12.5 MEDICAL MANAGEMENT

The treatment of children with cystic fibrosis has to encompass all the varied manifestations of the condition. Treatment is lifelong and careful, regular supervision is crucial for the child's optimum health. The older child and his family should understand the condition sufficiently to realize the importance of this. The aim of management is to enable the child to lead a normal life without undue dependence on others.

**Respiratory management**

Respiratory disease is usually the most serious aspect of cystic fibrosis and its seriousness often determines the child's prognosis. The main problems are thickened bronchial secretions and recurrent chest infections. Chest physiotherapy, bronchodilators and mucolytics help to loosen and liquefy the thickened secretions and also aid the prevention of infection. Antibiotics are used to eradicate infections that do occur.

Regular physiotherapy is probably the most important factor in managing respiratory problems. It clears secretions, helps to ventilate fully the lungs by teaching the child to breathe correctly and to maintain good posture, and it helps to keep the child fit and health. Chest physiotherapy consists of postural drainage, vibration and either percussion or forced expiration alternating with gentle diaphragmatic breathing. It should be performed at least twice a day. More frequent treatment may be necessary when the child has a chest infection. Ideally, the first treatment of the day should be after wakening to expel secretions which have accumulated overnight. All treatment should be performed before meals to reduce the risk of vomiting. Physiotherapy also includes a daily programme of 20–30 min of exercises such as swimming, running, skipping or cycling. Exercise increases fitness and muscle strength as well as helping to mobilize secretions.

Antibiotics may be used as a prophylactic measure, particularly during the first year of life. However, it is now more common to use antibiotics only when the child shows features of infection as prolonged use of antibiotics may encourage the development of resistant strains of bacteria. Children with cystic fibrosis need high doses of most antibiotics to penetrate their viscous secretions. For this reason, the intravenous route

**Table 12.1** Show the common antibiotics used intermittently in cystic fibrosis

| Organism | Antibiotic | Intravenous dose | Precautions |
|---|---|---|---|
| *Haemophilus influenzae* | Amoxycillin and | 50–100 mg/kg daily in divided doses | Observation for gastrointestinal side-effects and oral or peroneal thrush in infants due to alteration in normal flora |
| | Erythromycin | 25–50 mg/kg daily in divided doses | Contraindicated in those with biliary cirrhosis. Observe for mild allergic reactions – urticaria, skin rashes |
| Staphylococcus | Erythromycin | 25–50 mg/kg daily in divided doses | Contrindicated in those with biliary cirrhosis. Observe for mild allergic reactions – urticaria, skin rashes |
| *Pseudomonas aeruginosa* | Gentamycin and | 2.5–3 mg/kg 8 hourly | Serum levels monitored every 48 h to avoid side-effects of ototoxicity and nephrotoxicity |
| | Azlocillin | 75–100 mg/kg 8 hourly | Daily inspection of IV site for allergic reaction or venous thrombosis |

is preferred for intermittent antibiotic theraphy. Some children can have a permanent long, intravenous line inserted and they, or their parents, can be taught to give intravenous antibiotics as necessary; thus avoiding long periods of hospitalization. Aminoglycosides (gentamycin, tobramycin) are usually given by bolus injection, and penicillins and cephalosporins by infusion. Antibiotics may also be given by inhalation. Table 12.1 shows the common antibiotics used intermittently in cystic fibrosis.

**Nutritional management**

Optimum nutrition is essential in children with cystic fibrosis to prevent malnutrition and susceptibility to infection. The aims of dietary control are to maintain or increase weight and to promote growth.

Three factors cause the nutritional problems of the cystic fibrosis child:

- malabsorption due to pancreatic fibrosis;
- chronic respiratory infection causing breathlessness and increased sputum resulting in anorexia;
- increased basal metabolic rate.

Most children with cystic fibrosis can have a normal diet but the protein and calorie content should be increased. The increased basal metabolic rate means that the calorie intake of the cystic fibrosis child should be about 150% that of a normal child. A normal fat diet can be encouraged for most cystic fibrosis children to maintain a high calorie intake. A few children may develop steatorrhoea and abdominal discomfort when given fats and in such cases oils and fat derived from coconut oil may be better tolerated. Starchy foods in excess may also cause abdominal discomfort and flatulence. Babies can be breast fed or given standard modified cow's milk formulae. If a low fat preparation is required, 'Pregestimil' or a similar formula can be given.

Most cystic fibrosis children require pancreatic enzyme replacements which should be taken just before or during all meals and snacks (Table 12.2). The dosage of these preparations varies with the individual child. The optimum dose will reduce the size, frequency and consistency of the stools. Continued steatorrhoea is often due to very acidic gastric secretions which

**Table 12.2** Dosage and administration of common pancreatic enzyme supplements

| Pancreatic enzyme replacement | Preparation | Dose | Instructions |
|---|---|---|---|
| Pancrex V | Gelatin capsule containing powder | 0–12 months: 1–2 capsules/feed | Mix powder with a little milk and give on spoon |
| Creon | Enteric coated granules within a gelatin capsule | 1–3 years: ½–1 capsule/feed or meal | Open capsules and mix with fluid or food but do not let child chew as enteric coating is destroyed |
| | | 4–adulthood: 1–4 capsules/meal; 1 capsule/snack | Swallow whole before or during the meal or snack |
| Pancrease | Enteric coated granules within a gelatin capsule | 1–3 years: 1–2 capsules with each meal or snack | Mix granules with a little food or drink. Do not chew |
| | | 4–adulthood: 2–5 capsules/each meal; 1 capsule/snack | Swallow capsules whole before or during eating |

destroy the enzymes and may be helped by cimetidine given half an hour before meals.

As children with cystic fibrosis do not absorb fat well, they tend to be deficient in the fat soluble vitamins A, D, E and sometimes K. A multivitamin preparation in a water soluble form is given daily, at twice the dosage normally recommended for children. Vitamin E, 50–100 mg is given separately and oral vitamin K is also given to children who have a prolonged prothrombin time.

In the underweight child dietary supplements such as 'Build-up' can be given to increase calorie intake. Alternatively, 'Caloreen', which is a glucose powder, can be added to foods or drinks. Nasogastric or nasojejunal feeding can be performed overnight during chest infections when the child's weight loss is rapid and debilitating, and he is too ill to eat well.

**The future**

Heart-lung transplants may now become an option for those children whose lungs are severely affected by cystic fibrosis, providing there is no other complicating features such as biliary cirrhosis. Although a transplant will not cure the basic defect it does offer the child a longer life and potentially a better quality of life. Parents and adolescent patients may wish to discuss the possibility of a transplant and should be given the opportunity to do so.

12.6 NURSING CARE

**Assessment**

*Breathing*

- What is the child's rate and pattern of breathing?
- Does the child have a troublesome cough?
- What amount of sputum does the child produce daily? What colour and consistency is it?
- How often does the child have physiotheraphy? At what time(s) of day is this performed?

*Maintaining body temperature*

- Is the child pyrexial?

*Eating and drinking*

- Does the child have any dietary restrictions or supplements?
- What is his usual calorie intake?
- Which pancreatic enzyme supplements does he use? How does he prefer to take these?
- Does the child appear malnourished?

*Elimination*

- What are the child's normal bowel habits? What do his stools usually look like?
- Does he have problems with abdominal discomfort or distension?
- Does the child appear to perspire excessively?

*Communication*

- How much does the child and his family appear to understand about cystic fibrosis?
- How do they seem to have adjusted to the condition?

*Schooling*

- How does he receive his education? (Normal school, school for the handicapped, or by home tutor?)
- Has he missed much schooling due to illness?

*Mobility*

- What exercise does he normally do? Is this activity now affected by breathlessness?

*Expressing self-image*

- Does the child appear self-conscious about being underweight and underdeveloped for his age, or having a chronic cough and sputum?

## Dying

- Does this appear to be a particular fear at present for the child or his parents?

### Planning

To enable the child with cystic fibrosis to live a normal independent life he is only admitted to hospital when absolutely necessary and the length of hospitalization is kept to a minimum. Care at home also prevents the susceptible cystic fibrosis child from developing a hospital-acquired infection which may be antibiotic resistant.

The main role of the nurse is to teach the child and his parents how to manage the condition themselves and to offer psychological support (Table 12.3).

In hospital the child, who is usually admitted for treatment of a chest infection, may be nursed in a cubicle with protective precautions. If oxygen is required a low percentage should be used to prevent oxygen narcosis, a particular risk in children with long-standing obstructive airways disease. A long intravenous line may be inserted for the administration of antibiotics. The nurse should check the insertion site at least 4 hourly for any signs of local trauma. The child's temperature and the amount and characteristics of his sputum should be observed to monitor the effect of treatment. Salt supplements may be necessary if the pyrexia is prolonged.

If the child's mobility is restricted due to dyspnoea and intravenous therapy, he will need help with the daily activities of living. The undernourished child will need encouragement to change his position to prevent skin breakdown. Frequent washing may be required if the child perspires excessively. All care should be planned in liaison with the physiotherapist so that physiotherapy can be performed at the optimum time and frequency.

Parents are usually included in the child's treatment from the time of diagnosis and they should be allowed to be involved in as much of the child's care as possible. Hospitalization often provides an opportunity for the nurse to assess how the child and his parents have adjusted to the condition, and their ability to manage the various associated problems. Psychological problems related to the effects of chronic illness can be

**Table 12.3** Care plan for an adolescent with cystic fibrosis. Alan Carter, aged 15, has cystic fibrosis. He was diagnosed at the age of 18 months and has had a relatively trouble-free childhood. However, recently, according to his parents, he has been loathe to have physiotherapy and is not eating well. As a result, he has developed a chest infection and has lost weight. It is decided to admit him for a course of IV antibiotics and to encourage adequate nutrition. On admission, Alan is pyrexial and dyspnoeic and is obviously short and underweight for his age. His mother is particularly distressed by his deterioration

| Problem | Aim of care | Nursing intervention |
|---|---|---|
| Dyspnoea (resiratory rate 30) and increased sputum due to infection | For Alan to expectorate and to be able to breathe more easily | Administer prescribed nebulized bronchodilators and mucolytics ½ hour before physiotherapy<br>Plan physiotherapy 4 times daily in liaison with the physiotherapist<br>Administer prescribed antibiotics<br>Ensure clean sputum pot and tissues always available<br>Observe amount and characteristics of sputum<br>Observe respirations 4 hourly |
| Potential thrombophlebitis at site of IV cannula | For Alan's IV cannula site to remain patent | Use an aseptic technique for all IV drugs<br>Give prescribed IV anticoagulant following IV antibiotics<br>Observe cannula site 4 hourly for redness, swelling and pain |
| Pyrexia (temperature 38.5°C) | For Alan's temperature to drop to 37–37.2°C | Nurse Alan in a cool environment with minimal clothing<br>Provide a fan at the bedside<br>Record temperature 4 hourly |
| Underweight and malnourished due to anorexia | For Alan to maintain adequate nutrition and to gain 1 kg/week | Explain to Alan the importance of nutrition in the maintenance of health<br>Help Alan to choose a high calorie diet of his liking |

| Potential bulky stools and abdominal pain due to poor absorption of nutrients | For Alan to pass soft, formed stools without abdominal discomfort | Allow Alan to choose his own times for meals and snacks<br>Weigh Alan weekly<br>Record food refused/taken and daily calorie intake<br>Administer prescribed vitamins daily<br>Give prescribed enzyme replacements with every meal and snack<br>Observe the frequency/consistency/bulk of stools<br>Ask Alan to report any abdominal pain or distension |
|---|---|---|
| Resistance to treatment | For Alan to accept and comply with his treatment | Provide continuity of carers<br>Encourage Alan to talk about his feelings<br>Explain all treatment<br>Allow Alan as much independence and involvement in planning and implementing his care as possible<br>Encourage Alan to join other teenagers with cystic fibrosis<br>Record Alan's mood daily |
| Potential boredom due to hospitalization | For Alan to follow a normal level of activity | Allow Alan to carry out his normal routine for activities of daily living as far as possible<br>Allow time for Alan to continue his schooling/interests<br>Encourage visits from family and friends |
| Potential parental distress due to Alan's non-acceptance of his condition | For Alan's parents to recognize and explore their concerns | Allow parents time to talk about their feelings<br>Encourage Alan's parents to accept his need for privacy and independence<br>Encourage Alan and his parents to share their feelings |

particularly marked in the adolescent patient. Poor psychological adjustment to the condition often results in depression and poor compliance with treatment. Changes in family activities and the fear, anxiety and guilt felt by the parents can cause serious emotional problems and disruption for the whole family. Referral to a social worker or psychiatrist may be helpful to the child and his parents. The parents of the adolescent with cystic fibrosis need encouragement to allow him more independence and also to give him opportunity to share his feelings. When the adolescent is hospitalized the nurse should enable him to control his routine and treatment as far as possible but also be available to listen to his concerns. Where possible one nurse should be primarily allocated to the adolescent patient to facilitate the close relationship necessary for this sharing of feelings. The nurse should encourage her patient to include his family in such discussions. The adolescent may also benefit from a discussion group for other affected adolescents, where he can share his problems and anxieties with his peer group.

Hospitalization also provides an opportunity to assess the effect of the child's medical treatment. Respiratory function, dietary intake, weight and bowel habits should be monitored during the child's admission.

## 12.7 HEALTH EDUCATION

The healthier and fitter the cystic fibrosis child is, the less likely he is to succumb to chest infections. He can be helped to stay healthy by the following advice:

- To maintain a daily routine of medication, physiotherapy and exercise.
- Where possible to avoid close contact with others with known acute upper respiratory infections.
- To have immunizations against diptheria, tetanus, pertussis, poliomyelitis and measles. Pertussis and measles are liable to produce chest symptoms which may be very severe in the child with cystic fibrosis.
- To have influenza vaccine on an annual basis. Influenza can initiate or exacerbate chest infections.
- To take extra fluids and salt during febrile illnesses or during heatwaves.

- To avoid becoming overtired.
- To attend a cystic fibrosis clinic approximately 3-monthly (monthly during the first year of life) to provide careful and regular supervision, and early aggressive treatment of any infection.

The Cystic Fibrosis Research Trust helps and advises parents about the everyday problems of caring for a child with cystic fibrosis. This will help the parents to adopt a positive outlook and treat the affected child in the same way as his siblings. Acceptance of the condition by the family will help the affected child to come to terms with his condition and comply with its treatment.

# References and further reading

**Development of the respiratory tract**

Moore, K. (1977) *The Developing Human*, W.B. Saunders, Eastbourne

Nursing Times (1984) *Setting Up The Systems*, 11–13, Macmillan Journals, London

Wendell Smith, C.P. and Williams, P.L. (1984) *Basic Human Embryology*, Pitman, London

**Anatomy and physiology of the respiratory tract**

Godfrey, S. and Baum, J.D. (1979) *Clinical Paediatric Physiology*, Blackwell Scientific Publications, Oxford

**Assessment of the child with a respiratory problem**

Colley, J.R.T., Holland, W.W. and Corkhill, R.J. (1973) Influence of passive smoking and parental phlegm on pneumonia and bronchitis in early childhood. *Lancet*, **ii**, 1031–4

Durie, M. (1984) Respiratory problems and nursing intervention, *Nursing*, **2** (28) 826

Harlop, S. and Davies, A.M. (1974) Infant admissions to hospital and maternal smoking. *Lancet*, **i**, 529–32

Ogilvie, C. (1983) Dyspnoea, *BMJ*, **286**, 160

Roper, N. (1976) *Clinical Experience in Nurse Education*. Churchill Livingstone, Edinburgh

Roper, N., Logan, W.W. and Tierney, A.J. (1985) *The Elements of Nursing*, Churchill Livingstone, Edinburgh

Taylor, D.L. (1985) Assessing breathing sounds, *Nursing*, **15** (3) 60

**Respiratory therapy**

Glover, D. and Glover, M. (1978) *Respiratory therapy*, C.V. Mosby, St Louis

Hopkins, S.J. (1986) *Drugs and Pharmacology for Nurses*, Churchill Livingstone, Edinburgh

Nursing Times (1979) *Scan: Respiratory Function*, Macmillan Journals, London

Webber, B.A. (1980) *The Brompton Hospital Guide to Chest Physiotherapy*, Blackwell Scientific Publications, Oxford

**Respiratory distress syndrome**

Chinn, C. (1985) A baby with respiratory distress syndrome, *Nursing Times*, **81** (12) 31–6

Few, B.J. (1987) Neonatal update: surfactant replacement therapy, *The American Journal of Maternal Child Nursing*, **12**, 129

Greenough, A. and Roberton, N.R.C. (1985) Morbidity and survival in neonates ventilated for the respiratory distress syndrome, *BMJ*, **290**, 597–600

**Bronchiolitis**

Sims, D.F. (1979) Acute bronchiolitis in infancy, *Nursing Times*, **75** (43) 1842

Editorial (1980) Bronchiolitis in infancy and childhood, *BMJ*, **280**, 428

**Whooping cough**

Britten, N. and Wadsworth, J. (1986) Long-term respiratory sequelae of whooping cough in a nationally representative sample, *BMJ*, **292**, 441–4

Johnson, I.D.A., Hill, M., Anderson, H.R. and Lambert, H.P. (1985) Impact of whooping cough on patients and their families, *BMJ*, **290**, 1636–8

Simpson, H. (1987) Management of whooping cough, *Maternal and Child Health*, **12** (6) 168–71

Williams, W.O. *et al.* (1985) Respiratory sequelae of whooping cough, *BMJ*, **290**, 1937–40
Williams, W.O. (1987) The epidemiology of whooping cough, *Maternal and Child Health*, **12** (2) 40–3

**Asthma**

Chung, K.F. and Barnes, P.J. (1987) Treatment of asthma, *BMJ*, **294**, 103
Harrington, V.E. (1985) Philip: an asthmatic child, *Nursing*, 1 (6) 273–7
Hek, G.A. (1987) Patient education, *Professional Nurse*, 2 (6) 168
Price, R. (1985) Asthma in the family, *Nursing Times*, **81** (29) 24–6
Price, R. (1985) Peter and Paul, *Nursing Times*, **81** (29) 27–8
Rees, J. (1987) ABC of 1–7 bronchial asthma, *BMJ*, **294**, 753

**Croup and epiglottitis**

Levin, D.L. (1984) *A Practical Guide to Pediatric Intensive Care*, C.V. Mosby, St Louis

**Pneumonia**

Mok, J. (1982) Pneumonia in childhood, *Maternal and Child Health*, **7** (7) 264
Pinney, M. (1981) Pneumonia, *Am. J. Nursing*, **81** (3) 517

**Cystic fibrosis**

Carswell, F. (1986) Cystic fibrosis, *Br. J. Nurses in Child Health*, **1**, 6, 174–7
Goodchild, M.C. and Dodge, J.A. (1985) *Cystic fibrosis – Manual of Diagnosis and Management*, Ballière Tindall, London
Landau, L.I. (1987) Cystic fibrosis, *Medicine*, **2**, 1513–17
McKendrick, O.M. and Heaf, D. (1987) Coping with childhood death from cystic fibrosis, *Maternal and Child Health*, **12** (3) 72–8
Stullenbarger, B., Norris, J., Edgil, A.E. and Prosser, M.J. (1987) Family adaptation to cystic fibrosis, *Paediatric Nursing*, **13**, 29–31

# Index

| LIBRARY | SCHOOL OF NURSING |
|---------|-------------------|
| CLASS | |
| ACC No | |
| DATE | |
| PRICE | |